Two week loan

WITHDRAWN

Please return on or before the last
date stamped below.
Charges are made for late return.

2 1 APR 1997		
CANCELLED		

Community Mental Health Centers and the Courts

This important new book explores ways in which the mental health professions can assist the legal system in distributing justice more equitably, more quickly, and less expensively. In recent years, mental health professionals have been accused of helping criminals to "beat the rap" through findings of insanity or incompetence to stand trial. In fact, this book argues, the usual practice of administering pretrial evaluations in maximum-security hospitals has often infringed upon defendants' rights and proved costly to taxpayers.

The authors present a strong case for offering forensic mental health services on an outpatient basis in community mental health centers staffed by specially trained personnel. A pilot project incorporates community-based forensic services in Virginia, which led to legislation there, showed such services to be substantially less expensive and of better quality than those offered by hospitals. The Virginia project can serve as a model for other states. This book, containing comprehensive evaluations of those studies, is the first to discuss ways of dealing with practical problems (including political ones) in implementing the community-based system. It also adds significantly to knowledge about the nature and frequency of community mental health center interaction, about the forensic expertise of general clinicians, and about judges' understanding of mental health issues.

Gary B. Melton is a professor of psychology and law at the University of Nebraska–Lincoln. Lois A. Weithorn is an assistant professor of psychology at the University of Virginia. Christopher Slobogin is an associate professor of law at the University of Florida.

By Gary B. Melton,

Lois A. Weithorn, and

Christopher Slobogin

University of Nebraska Press: Lincoln and London

Community Mental Health Centers and the Courts
An Evaluation of Community-Based Forensic Services

The paper in this book meets
the guidelines for permanence
and durability of the Committee
on Production Guidelines for
Book Longevity of the Council
on Library Resources.

Library of Congress Cataloging
in Publication Data

Melton, Gary B.
Community mental health
centers and the courts.

Bibliography: p.
Includes index.
1. Community mental health
services – Law and
legislation – United States.
I. Weithorn, Lois A., 1953–
II. Slobogin, Christopher, 1951–
III. Title.
KF3828.M43   1985
344.73′0322   84-25751
ISBN 0-8032-3083-4
(alk. paper) 347.304322

Contents

Acknowledgments

A research and service project of the scope described in this volume inevitably depends on the cooperation and assistance of scores of groups and individuals. At the risk of errors of omission, we would like to acknowledge some of those who have contributed to the successful completion of the project.

The work described herein was supported by a grant from the Virginia Department of Mental Health and Mental Retardation. The department not only provided the finances for the project but also showed an unusual commitment to research and innovation in forensic mental health. A number of staff in the department's central office gave considerable time to the project (e.g., generating admissions data), but we wish to acknowledge particularly former commissioner Leo E. Kirven, Jr., present commissioner Joseph J. Bevilacqua, and the director of forensic services, Joel Dvoskin, for their ongoing support. Similar administrative support came from the office of the attorney general (Paul A. Sinclair and Maston T. Jacks) and the state Supreme Court (Robert N. Baldwin). The eighteen judges, commonwealth's attorneys, and defense attorneys who served on the project's advisory committee were crucial in the implementation of the project.

The project was initiated while all of us were on the faculty of the Institute of Law, Psychiatry and Public Policy at the University of Virginia. We wish to thank our colleagues, past and present, in the institute for their continuing consultation and collegiality. In particular, the institute's director, Richard J. Bonnie, and associate director, John Monahan, provided consistent support for the research and frequently acted as sounding boards for ideas.

The staffs of the participating community mental health centers gave considerable time to the project. We are especially grateful to the forensic teams in each of the demonstration clinics for their enthusiasm for the project and cooperation in the research. Thanks are also due the American Academy of Forensic Psychology and the American Academy of Judicial Education for their participation in data collection. The staff of the forensic unit at Central State Hospital were also very helpful in the collection of data in several of the studies reported in this book as well as in the implementation of the project as a whole.

We owe special thanks to Sue Lewis, the administrator of the Central State forensic unit, and James Dmitris, clinical director of the unit, for their continuing assistance.

A number of leaders in forensic mental health reviewed the test of forensic knowledge discussed in chapter 3: Walter Bromberg; Park Elliott Dietz; Newton L. P. Jackson, Jr.; Herbert Modlin; John Monahan; Bruce Dennis Sales; and John Torrens. Thanks are also due several Virginia judges and attorneys for their comments on the section of the exam on Virginia law.

Over the course of the project, our graduate research assistants in the psychology department at the University of Virginia included Kiki Litzie, Yorlunza Price, and Eric Vernberg. We acknowledge their assistance in data collection and analysis. Debra Mundie and Cathleen Oslzly provided able clerical assistance.

John Monahan reviewed the entire manuscript, and John Petrila read and commented on several chapters. Mr. Petrila, in his former position as director of forensic services in Missouri, and Marthagem Whitlock, director of forensic services in Tennessee, also generously gave of their time and expertise as we were developing the project.

Finally, we should note that the opinions expressed in the volume are our own and do not necessarily represent the position of the Department of Mental Health and Mental Retardation or the Institute of Law, Psychiatry and Public Policy.

Chapter 1

The Case for a Community-Based
Program of Forensic Services

The involvement of mental health professionals in the criminal justice system is clearly a matter of continuing controversy that peaks periodically in highly publicized cases. There is a widespread perception by the public (Pasewark & Seidenzahl, 1980) and by lawmakers (Pasewark & Pantle, 1979) that, whether unwittingly or through misplaced liberal zeal, mental health professionals often aid and abet vicious criminals in their attempts to "beat the rap" through a finding of incompetency to stand trial or insanity. Although such perceptions are often far from the objective reality (e.g., the number of successful insanity defenses tends to be grossly overestimated), the perceived reality may have substantial adverse political consequences for the mental health professions (cf. Melton, in press) and for public confidence in the courts. Even if people are often misinformed, public debate continues concerning the proper interaction between the mental health and criminal justice systems. At the same time, there has been considerable debate by scholars (e.g., Bonnie & Slobogin, 1980; Morse, 1978, 1982b) about whether mental health professionals' opinions are sufficiently relevant, reliable, and valid to merit attention in criminal cases.

Most of this debate has revolved around the *standards* by which mental health testimony is admitted and by which it is judged relevant. Much less attention has been directed toward the *procedures* by which mental health professionals' opinions are to be formulated and conveyed. However, given that there is little reason to believe that the need for such opinions is likely to disappear,[1] the process by which the delivery of forensic services[2] takes place is a matter of

---

1. Competency to stand trial is basic to due process, and the parties are obligated to raise the issue whenever there is a question of the defendant's competency. Drope v. Missouri, 420 U.S. 162 (1975); Pate v. Robinson, 383 U.S. 375 (1966). Hence, the need for information on this question is likely to persist. Similarly, although there has been a move to reform insanity laws, these reforms have most commonly consisted of adoption of a supplementary guilty but mentally ill verdict, not outright abolition of the insanity defense. Therefore, there is likely to be continued need for evidence on the insanity question.

2. As used in this volume, *forensic services* include any provision of services by mental health professionals to the legal system. This definition includes the provision of treatment for mentally disordered offenders. However, our discussion will be focused largely on forensic *evaluation*.

substantial importance. How might forensic services be organized to maximize the probability that the services provided will offer optimal assistance to the legal system? This book is directed toward an understanding of such systemic and procedural issues. Specifically, much of the book will focus on a series of studies we conducted of the interaction between the mental health system and the courts during the process of adoption of a system of community-based forensic services in Virginia. Before discussing alternative models of forensic service delivery, we review the nature of the assistance that mental health professionals are asked to provide to the legal system.

The Nature of Forensic Mental Health Services

The points of interaction between the mental health and the criminal justice system can conveniently be summarized by examining the steps in the criminal process at which they arise. (For a comprehensive review of the state of the art in forensic assessment and the nature of the questions raised, see Melton, Petrila, Poythress, & Slobogin, in press.) Prior to trial, questions posed to mental health professionals are likely to involve issues related to the degree to which the defendant might competently make decisions about his or her case.[3] Although the issue may involve competency to make a specific decision (e.g., competency to confess, plead guilty, represent oneself, or waive an insanity defense; see Melton et al., in press, chap. 5), the most common pretrial question—indeed the most common forensic question generally—concerns the defendant's competency to stand trial (i.e., whether the defendant has the ability to understand the nature of the proceedings against him and to assist counsel in his own defense;[4] see Melton et al., in press, chap. 4). At the adjudication phase, mental health professionals may be asked to address the defendant's mental state at the time of the offense (see Melton et al., in press, chap. 6), specifically whether the defendant was so mentally disordered that his conduct should be excused (insanity) or was unable to form the intent (mens rea) element of the offense or was in such an altered state of consciousness that his act was involuntary (automatism).

Finally, after conviction, mental health professionals may be asked to participate in a presentence evaluation. Such an evaluation might be part of a general presentence investigation, or it might be pursuant to a hearing on whether the

3. The question of competency to stand trial may arise at any point in the criminal process; see supra note 1. However, it is most commonly raised prior to trial.
4. Dusky v. United States, 363 U.S. 162 (1960).

death penalty should be levied or the defendant fits into a statutorily defined special offender status (e.g., mentally disordered sex offender, habitual offender, youthful offender). Regardless of the context, however, a presentence evaluation is likely to focus on culpability (e.g., whether the offense was "out of character" and an isolated, overdetermined event; whether mitigating or aggravating circumstances were present), amenability to treatment, or dangerousness (see Melton et al., in press, chap. 7).

Insofar as mental health professionals can offer assistance to the fact finder in decision making, it is important that the conditions under which the evaluation takes place facilitate the development of as much valid information as possible. This general concern is particularly acute with respect to competency to stand trial. Fundamental fairness demands that a defendant not be tried in de facto absentia. That is, it is basic to due process that a defendant not be tried when he is "not really there" and therefore unable to participate actively in his own defense. Accordingly, it is well established that courts have an obligation to consider the defendant's competency whenever it may be in question.[5] Similarly, at the adjudication phase, both the state and the defendant have substantial interest in avoiding the conviction of a morally blameless defendant (Monahan, 1973).[6] Finally, at sentencing, the consequences of an ill-advised decision are obvious, especially where the death penalty or a long prison sentence is an option.

These questions of forensic *evaluation* are, therefore, of great legal and moral importance in themselves. The involvement of the mental health system in the criminal justice system does not end with evaluation, however. At each of the points in the process, a positive finding might result in the defendant's commitment to a mental health facility (although, as we shall see, not necessarily one in the state department of mental health) for *treatment*, often of indefinite duration. The defendant who is found to be incompetent to stand trial, for example, will usually be committed for treatment to restore him or her to competency. Although the period of commitment cannot constitutionally exceed a period reasonably long enough to determine whether the defendant will be restored to competency within the foreseeable future,[7] many jurisdictions have not yet established procedures to ensure that commitment does not exceed constitutional limits (Roesch & Golding, 1979). Similarly, a defendant found not guilty by reason of insanity may be committed until such time as he or she is no longer mentally disordered and dangerous, even if the "dangerous" act which brought the defendant to the attention of authorities was no more serious than at-

5. *See supra* note 1.
6. *See* Whalem v. United States, 346 F.2d 812, 818–19 (D.C. Cir. 1965).
7. Jackson v. Indiana, 406 U.S. 715 (1972).

4

tempted shoplifting.[8] As a result of a sentencing proceeding, an offender may be subject to treatment under special conditions of confinement or as a condition of probation. Finally, once imprisoned, an inmate may be transferred to a mental health facility if it is felt that the inmate's needs for mental health treatment cannot be adequately met in the jail or prison.

As might be predicted from examination of the range of interaction between the mental health and criminal justice systems, the frequency of movement of offenders[9] from one system to the other is substantial. A recent national survey (Steadman, Monahan, Hartstone, Davis, & Robbins, 1982) showed an annual rate of hospitalization of 20,000 offenders. Although this figure is rather remarkable, it represents only a minority of offenders who enter the mental health system each year. The Steadman study only identified offenders committed for treatment as a result of an adjudication of a special status (e.g., incompetent to stand trial, insanity acquittee). Defendants referred for evaluation were not included. Application of findings by Steadman and colleagues of the incidence of commitment for *restoration of competency* to reviews of studies of the proportion of defendants referred for *evaluation of competency* who are actually found incompetent suggests that as many as 25,000 competency evaluations are performed each year. Steadman et al. (1982) also did not include persons who, as a result of involvement in the criminal justice system, are referred for outpatient mental health treatment. Although statistics are not available, it is possible that this is the largest class of offenders who enter the mental health system. Their data also do not cover the frequency of mental health involvement in the legal system arising from civil matters (e.g., child custody disputes).

The intrinsic significance and the frequency of involvement of mental health professionals in the legal system demand attention to the development of high-quality forensic services. Considerations in evaluating whether such services are adequately meeting the needs posed by the legal system include such factors as the effectiveness of the service delivery system (i.e., whether valid evaluations are performed, whether treatment is effective), the timeliness and fiscal costs of services, and the level of protection of defendants' rights. States have adopted a variety of models of forensic services; the variance in addressing the factors in the efficacy of forensic services is equally wide. We turn then to a description of current models of forensic services.

8. Jones v. United States, 103 S.Ct. 3043 (1983).
9. We use the label "offenders" for convenience. However, it does not properly apply to defendants referred for evaluation or found incompetent to stand trial (neither class having been yet convicted of a crime) or defendants found not guilty by reason of insanity (who were not found to be culpable).

Models of Forensic Service Systems

In general, forensic service systems can be classified according to where they lie on two dimensions: the level of restrictiveness (i.e., the degree of invasion of the offender's liberty) and the degree of integration of forensic services into the mental health system. With respect to the former dimension, the most restrictive means of provision of forensic services, a special maximum-security hospital, is also the traditional and most common form of forensic services. Typically, within such a model, a state has one or two special facilities that perform all or most forensic services. Frequently, the physical plant of such a hospital differs minimally from a correctional facility. Often overcrowding and distance to the central facility result in delays in defendants' being evaluated and then picked up; hence, the restrictiveness is exacerbated by length of hospitalization.

Next, and less restrictive, are regional forensic hospitals. States adopting such a model (e.g., Missouri; see Petrila, 1982) typically establish forensic centers within regional "civil" hospitals. Although services may still be provided on an inpatient basis, transportation costs are reduced, and there is greater access to the defendant's attorney, friends, and family than a central hospital would provide. Also, regional centers are frequently less forbidding and intrusive than hospitals specifically designed to house offenders.

The least restrictive model involves the delivery of forensic services in the community. In such a model, services are typically delivered on an outpatient basis in the jail or the clinic.

Except for states that provide all public forensic services in a special hospital, a mixed model with respect to level of restrictiveness is common. In a given jurisdiction, most evaluations may be performed in community clinics, but insanity acquittees may be treated in a special forensic hospital. Also, some outpatient evaluations may take place in clinics located at central or regional forensic facilities. For example, all state forensic evaluations in Michigan must by statute[10] be performed at the Center for Forensic Psychiatry, a forensic hospital located near Ann Arbor. However, the center conducts many of its competency evaluations on an outpatient basis.

On the second dimension concerning integration of forensic services, models of services may be differentiated by how "special" and isolated they are from other mental health services. At one extreme are forensic hospitals admin-

---

10. Mich. Comp. Laws. Ann. §§ 330.1128, 330.2026, 330.2028, and 330.2050 (1980), and § 768.20a (1982).

istered, at least in part, by the state Department of Corrections (e.g., Bridge-water State Hospital in Massachusetts). At a middle level are regional or community facilities that operate outside the regular mental health system. Ohio, for example, has established a network of community forensic programs, all of which are administratively unconnected with community mental health services even though they are funded by the state Department of Mental Health and Mental Retardation (Beran & Toomey, 1979b). The court clinics operated in some states (e.g., Massachusetts) are also exemplary of this middle level.

At the other end of the continuum are forensic services operated as part of regular mental health services. Thus, Tennessee provides some forensic services in its community mental health centers (Laben, Kashgarian, Nessa, & Spencer, 1977; Laben & Spencer, 1976); a similar model adopted by Virginia[11] is examined in detail in this book. Within hospital-based systems, the least special forensic services would be those operated as part of regular inpatient services without segregating persons admitted from the criminal justice system.

The Rationale for Community-Based Services

The previously cited literature gives substantial support for community-based services. Less persuasively, there is also reason to support services that are relatively highly integrated into the regular mental health system (i.e., community mental health centers). Both of these conclusions are especially pertinent to forensic evaluation, and our review therefore will focus on evaluation services. However, as we point out, many of these considerations apply as well to treatment of offenders. Although the least restrictive alternative for forensic treatment may frequently be an inpatient setting, within this stricture we would support services that are relatively unrestrictive and integrated into the regular mental health system. Beginning, though, where the case is clearest (i.e., with respect to evaluation), we will examine the high social and economic costs of the traditional forensic hospital system.

AVOIDING COSTS TO THE DEFENDANT

Undue Infringement on Liberty. The preservation of liberty is, of course, a fundamental interest. Where the state seeks to infringe on liberty, it must do so as parsimoniously as possible to meet the compelling state purpose—that is, the intervention must be no more restrictive than is required to meet the state's

11. See Va. Code § 19.2-169.5(B) (Cum. Supp. 1982).

interest. Applying this principle to forensic mental health, the Supreme Court has held that "at the least, due process requires that the nature and duration of commitment bear some reasonable relation to the purpose for which the individual is committed."[12] Thus, several commentators have argued that unnecessary hospitalization (especially hospitalization under conditions of maximum security) violates the defendant's right to be evaluated and treated in the least restrictive environment (Janis, 1974; Steinberg, 1978; Winick, 1983; see also American Bar Association, 1983, Stds. 7-4.3, 7-4.9[a], 7-7.2[b], and 7-7.16, and commentary). The state's interest in avoiding the trial of an incompetent person may justify a requirement that the defendant submit to an evaluation if his or her competency is in question;[13] it does not, however, justify hospitalization if the evaluation could be performed in the community.

Detention without Bail. The eighth amendment tersely provides that "excessive bail shall not be required." Thus, the Constitution is ambiguous as to the situations under which the opportunity to post bail is required. This unclarity has been reduced, however, by state constitutional provisions[14] and case law (for a summary, see Department of Justice, 1983, pp. 58–59). The Supreme Court has identified three purposes for bail: the provision of bail assists the defendant by increasing his ability to prepare for his defense; it prevents de facto punishment through incarceration without a conviction; it gives meaning to the presumption of innocence.[15] Indeed, it is arguable that the deprivation of bail is justifiable only if such action is necessary to ensure the defendant's presence at trial (ABA, 1983, commentary about Std. 7-4.3; Tribe, 1970). However, when a defendant is required to submit to an inpatient evaluation in a secure facility, it results in de facto detention without bail. Particularly given the prosecution's ability to compel a competency evaluation, there is the risk of abuse of the forensic mental health system to confine a defendant who would otherwise be able to post bail.

Attenuation of the Right to a Speedy Trial. The sixth amendment accords the right to a speedy trial. This right differs from other procedural rights preserved for criminal defendants by the Bill of Rights because it is based on the interests

12. Jackson v. Indiana, 406 U.S. 715, 737 (1972). *See also* Shelton v. Tucker, 364 U.S. 479, 488 (1960) (noting the least restrictive alternative doctrine); Lake v. Cameron, 364 F.2d 657 (D.C. Cir. 1966) (applying the LRA concept to mental health law).

13. Issues with respect to the state's compulsion of a competency evaluation are reviewed by Slobogin (1982, especially pp. 87–94).

14. Forty state constitutions provide a right to bail (Whitebread, 1980, § 17.01).

15. Stack v. Boyle, 342 U.S. 1, 4 (1951).

of society (apart from whatever interest the state has in ensuring fair treatment of the defendant) as well as of defendants themselves. Indeed, defendants who are able to post bail may frequently find it to their advantage to *delay* trials (Swigert & Farrell, 1980); adverse community sentiment may abate in the meantime, and prosecuting witnesses may become unavailable. In *Barker v. Wingo,*[16] the Supreme Court noted several reasons why a speedy trial is in society's interests: delays in trials contribute to the backlogs in the courts, which result in increased use of plea bargaining and manipulation of the justice system by defendants; the defendant who is awaiting trial has the opportunity to commit other crimes; the opportunity to jump bail may become more inviting the longer the defendant is free on bail; the delay between arrest and punishment may decrease the probability of rehabilitation; if the defendant is unable to post bail, lengthy pretrial periods result in more jail overcrowding, increased costs, and loss of wages that the defendant might be earning.[17]

Nonetheless, the defendant also may have substantial interest in a speedy trial. The guarantee by the sixth amendment is designed "to prevent undue and oppressive incarceration prior to trial, to minimize anxiety and concern accompanying public accusation and to limit the possibilities that long delay will impair the ability of an accused to defend himself."[18] Lengthy and needless inpatient confinement arguably infringes on such a right. However, it should be noted that the courts have been loath to extend the constitutional right to a speedy trial, in part because the only remedy is outright dismissal of the charges.[19] Moreover, the Federal Speedy Trial Act of 1974 explicitly exempts the time spent in competency evaluations from the time that is computed in setting a deadline for the beginning of the trial.[20] Nonetheless, the point here is that confinement for forensic evaluation adversely affects interests of constitutional proportion.

Stigma. A defendant confined for forensic evaluation may possibly acquire the stigma of being a mental patient (see Goffman, 1961; Goldstein, 1979; McEwen, 1980). The Supreme Court has recognized this fact in holding that prisoners have a right to the rudiments of procedural due process in decisions concerning transfer from a correctional institution to a mental hospital.[21] So even though the prisoner has already lost his or her liberty, there is a residual interest in avoiding

16. 407 U.S. 514 (1972).

17. *Id.* at 519–21.

18. Barker v. Wingo, 407 U.S. 514, 532 (1972); Smith v. Hooey, 393 U.S. 374, 378 (1969); United States v. Ewell, 383 U.S. 16, 120 (1966); *see also* United States v. McDonald, 102 S.Ct. 1497, 1502 (1982).

19. *See* Barker v. Wingo, 407 U.S. 514, 522 (1972).

20. 18 U.S.C.A. § 3161(h)(1) (1982).

21. Vitek v. Jones, 445 U.S. 480 (1980).

the stigma of mental hospitalization and the invasion of privacy inherent in forced treatment. Accordingly, there is a cognizable loss of liberty and privacy from the fact of hospitalization per se; defendants have a special interest, therefore, in avoiding inpatient evaluations whenever possible.

Difficulty in Trial Preparation. An adversary system requires that both sides be able to present their cases in the best light (Thibaut & Walker, 1978). Denial of such a right is especially egregious for criminal defendants because of our strong desire to avoid erroneous convictions and to preserve perceived justice in the criminal law because of its meaning for the defendant and the community. Consequently, this interest is embedded in the due process clause of the fifth and fourteenth amendments and the right to effective assistance of counsel under the sixth amendment. In some cases, the defendant's ability to prepare his case effectively may be impaired because of his confinement.[22] There may be compelling reasons in many cases, nonetheless, to incarcerate a defendant who is awaiting trial (e.g., the probability of a defendant's failing to appear at trial; incarceration as punishment for an offense for which the defendant has already been convicted and sentenced). Again, it is arguable that *unnecessary* incarceration before trial (as in unnecessary hospitalization) is an unconstitutional interference with the defendant's ability to assist in the preparation of a defense. Such an argument would be particularly potent in instances where the defendant exercises the right to self-representation.[23]

AVOIDING COSTS TO THE STATE

The Costs of Inpatient Care. When the state hospitalizes a defendant who would otherwise be free on bail, the state is assuming a substantial financial commitment. Moreover, given the cost of treatment programs, we would expect that the cost of hospitalization would exceed the cost of maintaining a defendant in the jail if the defendant is not able to post bail. Because of the frequency of forensic evaluations, these added costs are far from trivial. In Virginia, for example, the cost per day for hospitalization is $85 versus a per diem cost for jail of $15. (The full cost analysis is presented in chapter 2; see also Laben et al., 1977, for a comparison of the costs of inpatient versus community-based forensic services in Tennessee.) A hospitalization of more than a month is com-

---

22. The Supreme Court has recognized that "if a defendant is locked up, he is hindered in his ability to gather evidence, contact witnesses, or otherwise prepare his defense." Barker v. Wingo, 407 U.S. 514, 533 (1972). The interest in avoiding such hindrance of the defense is "the most serious [interest of defendants in a speedy trial] . . . because the inability of a defendant adequately to prepare his case skews the fairness of the entire system." *Id.* at 532.

23. *See* Faretta v. California, 422 U.S. 806 (1975).

10

mon for competency evaluations in states relying on a central forensic hospital (see, e.g., Laben et al., 1977; McCall, 1979).

The Costs of Transportation. In states with a central forensic hospital, considerable costs can be accrued in transporting defendants to the hospital from remote counties. The cost of the transportation itself is added to the cost of providing sheriff's deputies to escort the defendant. This cost can amount to several person-days in overtime (for example, two deputies may be required to transport a defendant to a hospital several hours away). In addition, replacements are needed for the deputies while they are away.

There are analogous costs for experts' travel. When a single facility serves a whole state, the psychiatrists and psychologists may find that they spend much of their time on the road, because they travel to give testimony in courts in distant counties. Such use of professionals' time is expensive and wasteful, particularly given the difficulties of attracting qualified professionals to work in state hospitals (see Stone, 1982).

Conditions for Abuse of the System. Another problem with an inpatient forensic system is that, despite the problems already mentioned, the existence of an inpatient system may invite frivolous evaluations. Referrals for evaluation of competency to stand trial are likely to be for reasons other than the question overtly presented (Roesch & Golding, 1978, 1980). This point is reflected in the gross overreferral of defendants for competency evaluations.[24] Because the competency evaluation represents a convenient ruse to remove the defendant from the community, there is considerable potential for misuse of an inpatient evaluation system at great cost to the defendant, the taxpayers, or both (ABA, 1983, Std. 7-4.2 and commentary). As already noted, prosecutors may raise the competency question to force incarceration without bail. They may also use the competency evaluation for de facto punishment of a defendant when the evidence may be too weak to obtain a conviction. Prosecutors may also perceive the forensic evaluation as a mechanism for discovery of information about the alleged offense outside the strictures that the fifth and sixth amendments place on police interrogation (cf. Slobogin, 1982). Although the latter abuse is not limited to inpatient evaluations, confinement over an extended period gives much more opportunity to obtain incriminating information than does an outpatient evaluation. The defense may also find the inpatient evaluation system attractive for illegitimate purposes. Notably, an inpatient evaluation may remove

24. No more than one in three—perhaps closer to one in ten—defendants referred for competency evaluations is actually found to be incompetent to stand trial (Melton et al., in press, § 4.06(a)).

the defendant from the community when adverse sentiment is highest and provide a means of delaying the proceedings. Judges are often aware of these abuses of the system, but typically they order the evaluation summarily because of the desire to be certain that the defendant is competent if one of the parties raises a question in that regard (Roesch & Golding, 1978).

IMPROVING THE QUALITY OF FORENSIC SERVICES
The cost of inpatient services might be justified if the validity of outpatient evaluations were lower. However, there is actually more reason to believe that community-based evaluations are likely to be at least equal and often *higher* in quality. Before reciting the evidence on this point, it may be useful to underline the significance of the availability of high-quality forensic services.

The Significance of Quality. The quality of forensic services may be a concern of both the prosecution and the defense. On the one hand, forensic services in the public sector are typically the primary source available to prosecutors for expert evidence on questions about the defendant's mental condition. The state, therefore, has an interest in ensuring that public forensic services are of high quality. On the other hand, indigent defendants may be unable to obtain private evaluations. As noted earlier in this chapter, questions of competency to stand trial and mental state at the time of the offense are of substantial importance in the pursuit of justice. The defense may benefit, however, not just from having expert evidence on questions actually adjudicated in the case. The defense is likely to be handicapped in the development of its strategy if it is unable to explore possible defenses. Besides the desirability of this exploration for planning strategy, exploratory evaluation often presents information about mitigating concerns which are useful in plea bargaining or at sentencing; indeed, the ultimate significance of forensic evaluation may be greatest at these points in the process (Hastings & Bonnie, 1981).

It seems inherently unjust in such circumstances to deprive indigent defendants of mental health expertise which is available to defendants who can afford it. Several courts (see also ABA, 1983, commentary about Std. 7-3.3) have in fact held that denial of access to mental health evaluations when indicated is a violation of the defendant's sixth-amendment right to effective assistance of counsel.[25] This conclusion might reasonably be extended to a right to forensic services of high quality. A poor evaluation is unlikely to result in demonstrable

25. *E.g.*, Ake v. Oklahoma, 53 U.S.L.W. 4179 (U.S. Feb. 26, 1985). Wood v. Zahradnick, 578 F.2d 980 (4th Cir. 1978); United States v. Edwards, 488 F.2d 1154, 1163 (5th Cir. 1974); People v. Frierson, 25 Cal. 3d 142, 599 P.2d 587, 158 Cal. Rptr. 281 (1979).

assistance. It may be functionally equivalent to a denial of access to mental health expertise. Although courts may be reluctant to exercise significant review over the content and process of forensic evaluation, it seems clear that the constitutional interest (if not outright protection) extends beyond the existence of forensic services to their quality.

Access to Key Informants. Given, then, the significance of high-quality forensic services, we return to the question of the relative merits of community-based and hospital-based systems. In that regard, superiority of community-based evaluation systems would be expected, simply because it is easier to do forensic evaluation and consultation in the community. Friends and relatives are more likely to be accessible for interviews to corroborate the defendant's story or a possible psychological formulation. Still more important, the referring attorney is more likely to be easily available. It is often helpful to review particular questions or theories that the attorney wishes addressed. If testimony is desired, preparation for testimony is easier when there is time to go over issues at some length face to face (see ABA, 1983, Std. 7-3.12[a] and commentary).

Also, an important part of forensic services is *consultation,* which is difficult to perform long-distance. This point is most clearly demonstrated with respect to competency to stand trial (see Melton et al., in press, chaps. 4 and 14). The nature of the issue is such that, at least in close cases, there is a real need to involve the defense attorney directly in the evaluation. The question of competency to stand trial involves the *interaction* between counsel and client; competency is not purely an internal attribute of the defendant. The defendant's ability to assist counsel in his or her own defense depends in part on the attorney's ability to work with a difficult client. Indeed, the unduly high frequency of competency referrals is probably not exclusively a problem of abuse of the system or ignorance of the standards, although these factors undoubtedly apply. Many referrals, when there is not really a question of the defendant's competency, may reflect an attorney's difficulty in working with a particular client. Such problems are not surprising because legal education typically includes little, if any, training in client interviewing and counseling. The frequency of inappropriate referrals may be reduced and the quality of administration of justice ultimately improved when forensic clinicians perceive consultation as part of their job and have access to attorneys to be able to perform such consultation.

Quality of Staff. Another reason that community-based forensic services are likely to be superior to inpatient services is that it has traditionally been difficult to attract qualified professionals to state hospitals (Stone, 1982). This problem may be particularly acute in state forensic units, which are often the least desirable facilities of all. The preponderance of foreign-born, foreign-trained physicians in state hospitals is well known (Torrey & Taylor, 1973). Often such clinicians have little formal psychiatric training, much less formal forensic training. Moreover, difficulties in communication because of lack of fluency in spoken English assume particular significance when understanding subtleties in a defendant's story may shape the legal fact finder's judgment of the defendant's mental state at the time of the offense, or when (as is usually the case with respect to competency to stand trial; see Roesch & Golding, 1978, 1980) the clinician's opinion is dispositive of the outcome. We do not mean to suggest, of course, that all forensic clinicians or even all foreign-born, foreign-trained forensic clinicians in state hospitals are unqualified. However, it does seem clear to us that the probability of attracting skilled clinicians to forensic work is higher in a community-based system.

Evaluation Research. Perhaps the most persuasive evidence for the probable quality of community-based forensic services is simply that ample empirical data indicate that most forensic evaluations can be performed in brief interviews without extended inpatient observation. Roesch and Golding (1980; Roesch, 1979) found that mental-status examinations at intake were good predictors of ultimate conclusions as to defendant's competency to stand trial at the end of their inpatient stay. They also found that trained laypersons' opinions formed during brief semistructured interviews were highly correlated with professionals' opinions formulated at the end of weeks of hospitalization (Roesch, 1978; Roesch & Golding, 1980). The high reliability and validity of brief competency evaluations has been demonstrated in several other studies (Golding, Roesch, & Schreiber, in press; Laboratory of Community Psychiatry, 1974; Poythress & Stock, 1980).

Evidence also shows that brief, semistructured interviews about mental state at the time of the offense can screen out many defendants who do not have a viable psychological defense without false negatives (i.e., errors in screening out defendants who ultimately are found to have been significantly mentally disordered at the time of the offense). In a study conducted as part of the Virginia project reported in this volume (Slobogin, Melton, & Showalter, 1984), such a result was obtained using an interview guide and decision tree (see appendix A). The clinicians did a brief interview, and they had no additional information available other than the charges pending against the defendant. Such a comprehensive evaluation (more extensive interviews and information gathering) for defendants screened in on the basis of the brief interview could

14

also be done in the community in most cases. Indeed, as already noted, such data gathering is usually done more easily in the community than in hospital settings.

In short, there is no empirical basis for a belief that forensic evaluations cannot be performed on an outpatient basis. To the contrary, there actually is some reason to believe that community-based services are likely to be superior in quality to hospital-based services. Aside from the costs of inpatient evaluations to both defendants (many of these costs involving infringement on constitutionally protected interests) and the state, an inpatient system cannot be justified without compelling evidence that inpatient evaluations are necessary to develop valid opinions about the defendant's mental condition.

There are analogous arguments with respect to forensic treatment services. The available outcome research suggests that hospitalization is rarely warranted for treatment (Kiesler, 1982a). For schizophrenics, a mix of phenothiazines and outpatient supports (e.g., day hospitals) is often as effective, or more effective, than inpatient services (see, e.g., Marx, Test, & Stein, 1973). For persons who are found to be incompetent to stand trial as a result of mental retardation, the special education about the legal process necessary to raise them to competency can usually be performed at least as effectively in the community as in an inpatient setting. Moreover, in many cases, there is not a clear public-safety interest in incarcerating a defendant while he or she is being treated following an adjudication of incompetency or insanity. In some jurisdictions, defendants who are found incompetent or insane often have not been charged with serious offenses (see, e.g., Petrila, 1982). When neither treatment needs nor public safety necessitate inpatient treatment, confinement (especially in a maximum-security facility) constitutes de facto punishment without a conviction and, therefore, a clear violation of constitutional due process.[26]

The Counterarguments

Even with this rather lengthy list of arguments in favor of community-based systems, there has been no rush by the states to develop community-based forensic services. We might speculate that the most powerful reason for this lack of reform has simply been institutional inertia. Although there is a certain resistance to change in any bureaucracy (cf. Reppucci & Saunders, 1983), such inertia is especially meaningful in the legal system. In a system based on

26. *See* O'Connor v. Donaldson, 422 U.S. 563 (1975); Jackson v. Indiana, 406 U.S. 715 (1972).

the principle of *stare decisis*,[27] policymakers may be easily persuaded by the rationale that "we do it that way because that's the way it's always been." Moreover, despite the contrary empirical evidence, the argument that longer observation (as in an inpatient evaluation) is more valid is intuitively appealing. In particular, some believe that lengthy inpatient evaluation is necessary to detect malingering. Such an argument overlooks these facts: investigation of a defendant's history is easier in the community, positive findings (e.g., insane, incompetent to stand trial) are reached with relatively small proportions of defendants, inconsistencies suggestive of malingering in a defendant's story can often be detected in a brief interview, and the time actually spent on evaluation may be a matter of hours in a month-long inpatient evaluation.

More persuasive counterarguments can be made. Even though community-based evaluations are potentially valid, systemic factors may block the development of a well-functioning community-based system of forensic services even when states are committed to adopting, or at least trying, a community-based model. Many community mental health centers are inadequately staffed to deliver forensic services. Rural centers often lack professionals who possess the doctoral-level credentials (Langsley & Robinowitz, 1979; Richards & Gottfredson, 1978) that many courts require for qualification as an expert (Dix & Poythress, 1981). There may not be a critical mass of cases of mentally disordered offenders in sparsely populated areas, so clinicians are unable to quickly "learn by doing." Also, even if the quality of services in a central hospital is poor, there is at least consistency and equity in application of services. Quality control becomes a problem in a decentralized system. These potential problems have led some authorities (e.g., Petrila, 1981) to suggest that, although the central-hospital model of forensic services should be abandoned in favor of less restrictive services, the optimal model is regional rather than community-based.

Both the benefits that attorneys now obtain from abusing the system and judges' reluctance to change might also lead to ineffectiveness of a community-based system. One result, for example, might be to use community services on a pro forma basis before sending defendants to the state hospital. Such circumvention of the system might also be engineered by community clinics themselves. Offenders are unattractive clients, and many mental health professionals dislike the scrutiny and confrontation that inevitably accompany forensic work. Although some mental health professionals probably enjoy the role of expert, at least as many are deterred from forensic work by the role conflicts it engenders and the prospect of cross-examination.

27. The principle of *stare decisis* refers to the principle that precedent is binding.

These hypothetical problems in the development of community-based forensic services are not inherent in community-based services; rather, they represent issues which deserve administrative attention in planning and implementation. Nonetheless, they may be sufficiently powerful that the success of community-based forensic services is far from inevitable. Although there is a strong
case to be made for community-based forensic services on the basis of analyses of the costs of hospital-based services and the potential quality of community-based services, there is still a need for careful evaluation research on the
effectiveness of community-based services when they are developed.

Previous Evaluation Research

Prior to the studies reported in this book, only two attempts had been made to
validate the effectiveness of community-based forensic services in the field.
Beran and Toomey (1979b) edited a volume reporting data from a demonstration project involving community forensic clinics in Ohio, and Laben and her
colleagues (Laben et al., 1977; Laben & Spencer, 1976) reported initial results
of decentralization of forensic evaluation services in Tennessee. We have also
examined more recent unpublished descriptive data from Tennessee (M. Whitlock, personal communication; reported in Forensic Evaluation Training and
Research Center, 1982). Although neither the Ohio nor the Tennessee evaluation was comprehensive, review of these projects is useful in setting the context
for the Virginia program.

OHIO

In response to a concern that the central forensic unit, Lima State Hospital
(LSH), was "overpopulated, understaffed, and very expensive" (Roth, 1979, p.
103), Ohio experimented with six community forensic centers under contract
from the state department of mental health. Although quantitative data were not
reported, referring judges and probation officers were said to have uniformly
reported that the new demonstration centers, all established by 1974, provided
generally better, more detailed, and more comprehensive reports than did LSH.
Center staff were described as more professional and courteous, and waiting
periods were reduced (Beran & Toomey, 1979a).

As a result of these initial positive findings, Ohio committed itself to a community-based system. However, some limitations of this system should be
noted. More important, the centers have generally been reluctant to perform
evaluations of competency to stand trial and mental state at the time of the

offense; rather, the system is geared toward presentence evaluations—evaluations that would not have been performed at LSH (Carlson, 1979). Thus, the primary effect at least of the pilot project may have been to "widen the net" of mental health and criminal justice interaction, not to reduce referrals to LSH. Moreover, there were indications that the pilot project staff frequently did not understand legal standards they were asked to address in evaluations (Beran & Toomey, 1979a).

TENNESSEE

In 1974 the Tennessee General Assembly enacted a statutory change enabling competency evaluations to be performed by staff at community mental health centers.[28] As reported by Laben and Spencer (1976), there was a dual impetus to the reform: cost of inpatient care and an attorney general's opinion about the significance of *Jackson v. Indiana*[29] for the Tennessee forensic service system. Laben and Spencer (1976) described the central forensic unit as having had the worst characteristics of such facilities:

In 1972, all of the staff wore white uniforms and all of the residents wore green, heavy cotton pajama outfits. All the walls had been painted beige white with no accent colors. The authors' impression was that for these people, the world was only green and white. There were no personal areas for residents' possessions, neither closets nor bedside stands. Most residents slept on iron bed frames chained to the walls. There were no individualized stalls or doors for the toilets. The lack of sufficient cooling equipment in hot weather and heat that could be adequately regulated in winter made living conditions often unbearable. Residents were not allowed access to the front yard inside the double chain link and barbed wire fence within guards' vision. They were allowed outdoors only onto two smaller courtyards. There were not a sufficient number of jackets or umbrellas to allow the residents to go to the smaller courtyards in inclement weather. Occupational and recreational budgets could, in the most generous opinions, only be called a pittance. (p. 406)

To make matters worse, these medieval conditions—certainly unduly restrictive[30] and inhumane—were expensive. The cost of hospitalization was exacerbated by delays in picking up defendants because of the distance that sheriffs were required to travel (e.g., 213 miles to Memphis, Tennessee's largest city) and by inadequate staffing which delayed completion of the evaluation.

28. Tenn. Code Ann. § 33-708 (Cum. Supp. 1982).

29. 406 U.S. 715 (1972). Tennessee was said to be in violation of *Jackson* because of unduly long commitments of incompetent defendants and overly restrictive conditions of confinement of forensic patients. *See* Laben et al. (1977); Laben & Spencer (1976).

30. *See supra* notes 12, 26, and 29, and accompanying text.

Thus, the median length of hospitalization for evaluation was more than forty days, despite court orders limiting the evaluation to thirty days.

As a result, a pilot project of community-based evaluations was undertaken in Memphis. The average cost of evaluation was reduced by two-thirds, and the length of time from referral to testimony was reduced from fifteen weeks to twenty-one days (Laben et al., 1977). After the success of the pilot project, twenty-three outpatient evaluation units were established. All initial evaluations are done in these community centers; about 20 percent of these defendants are ultimately hospitalized (M. Whitlock, personal communication). The number of evaluations performed has increased each year since the program's inception, again raising a question of net-widening and relative aggregate costs.

VIRGINIA

Like most states, Virginia relied for decades on maximum-security inpatient units for most forensic evaluations. Indeed, the forensic service system was sufficiently centralized that its entire scope could be easily summarized in one paragraph of the final report by the Commissioner's Committee (1982):

> For many years, the Department [of Mental Health and Mental Retardation] maintained two Forensic Units, one at Southwestern State Hospital at Marion and the other at Central State Hospital in Petersburg. Southwestern State admitted approximately 400 criminal defendants a year, while Central State admitted another 575 defendants a year. Each hospital provided pretrial evaluations . . . , principally on the issues of competency to stand trial and mental state at the time of the offense. Each hospital also provided treatment for defendants found incompetent to stand trial, those found not guilty by reason of insanity, those who required emergency treatment prior to trial, and prisoners transferred from the Department of Corrections. Together with some clinicians who occasionally performed evaluations in the community, these two hospitals constituted the entire forensic evaluation and treatment system in the State of Virginia until 1979. (p. 4)

The typical period of confinement for evaluation lasted more than a month (McCall, 1979), at the end of which a brief conclusory report was written (see chapter 4). The forensic service system thus relied on prolonged and unnecessary confinement of defendants for evaluations at great cost, with products of questionable quality.

Midst the various arguments for community-based services, the clear impetus for reform of the Virginia system was simply fiscal cost.[31] In fall 1979 the Department of Mental Health and Mental Retardation (DMHMR) was faced with

31. The events leading to the establishment and implementation of a demonstration program of community-based forensic services are described in detail in chapter 6.

the prospect of sizable budget cuts. Then-commissioner Leo Kirven, Jr., decided to achieve part of this budget reduction by transferring the forensic unit at Southwestern State Hospital to the Department of Corrections, a decision which was implemented in mid-1980.[32] This move was dramatic and forced the issue of the proper organization of forensic services. The prospect of overwhelming the Central State unit with referrals was in fact realized (Commissioner's Committee, 1982)—a situation that demanded consideration of alternative means of forensic service delivery.

DMHMR had been concerned for some time about unnecessarily high costs of forensic services. In the face of fiscal austerity, unnecessary inpatient forensic services in effect drained resources from civil mental health services. As an initial step, in 1977 DMHMR had begun contracting with the Institute of Law, Psychiatry and Public Policy at the University of Virginia for forensic training of community mental health professionals, partially in the hope that community mental health centers would begin assuming some of the responsibility for forensic services. There had been no active effort, however, to ensure that such an adjunct to the forensic hospitals developed. In other words, there were some DMHMR-sponsored continuing education workshops on forensic mental health issues, but prior to 1980 there was little effort to ensure that knowledge acquired in the workshops was translated into practice. No administrative action had been taken to implement a *system* of community-based forensic services. For example, there were no incentives for judges to refer defendants to community mental health centers or, for that matter, for the centers to offer such a service.

In the wake then of the closing of the forensic unit at Southwestern State and as the next logical step in the department's attempts to contain the costs of forensic evaluations, a pilot project of community-based forensic services was established by the Virginia General Assembly with the enactment of House Joint Resolution No. 22 in March 1980. H.J.R. 22, reprinted in full in appendix B, provided for the establishment of a Forensic Evaluation Training and Research Center (in fact established in the Institute of Law, Psychiatry and Public Policy) to train clinicians from community mental health centers in selected jurisdictions ("demonstration service projects") as forensic evaluators and to evaluate the program. The scope of the program was to include evaluations of competency

---

32. Ironically, the savings that DMHMR had expected most directly as a result of this transfer did not occur. The transfer of physical facilities to the Department of Corrections did not result in a transfer of all mental health services for prisoners, as apparently had been envisioned by DMHMR (Commissioner's Committee, 1982). Nonetheless, the substantially greater proportion of services threatened by the closing of the unit at Southwestern State was in evaluation of defendants, not in treatment of prisoners.

to stand trial and "other appropriate psychological evaluations for the court." By September 1982 a report was to be submitted to the General Assembly describing the impact of the program and presenting a plan, including proposals for statutory reform as needed, for statewide implementation of community-based forensic services.

Why Do a Pilot Project?

It is reasonable to ask why the pilot project envisioned in H.J.R. 22 was necessary. Why not just implement a statewide community-based system? Indeed, the General Assembly itself had concluded, in the "whereas" clauses of H.J.R. 22, that "the experiences of other states demonstrate that forensic evaluations of criminal defendants can be efficiently and competently performed by appropriately trained clinical personnel in community mental health clinics on an outpatient basis at less expense than in inpatient setting." Was there anything left to study?

This question was especially acute because the arbitrary selection for research of a few jurisdictions in which to try community-based forensic services potentially raised issues of equal protection. Without regard to their personal characteristics (other than the county or city in which they had been charged with a crime), some defendants would be assigned to the project for evaluation, while others would have the substantially more intrusive hospital-based evaluations. Thus, the usual questions were raised about the probability of sufficient new knowledge to warrant investment of resources in a study. The significance of these issues was intensified by the prospect of disparities in the type of evaluation accorded defendants, when those disparities were based on experimental conditions alone. Such equal protection issues often make experiments[33] in the legal system ethically and legally unjustifiable (Federal Judicial Center, 1981). It seems manifestly unjust, for example, to base a defendant's sentence on the luck of assignment to one or another experimental condition.

In this instance, however, the Virginia legislature's decision to initiate a pilot project was wise for several reasons. First, practical and political realities made statewide implementation unfeasible. It was simply not possible to do the necessary training and local coordination to put the program into place in all court districts at once. Even if it had been possible (as it might be in a geographically small state with adaptable organizational structures for interaction between the

33. As used here, the term *experiment* does not refer to innovation per se. Rather, it is a technical term denoting research in which there is random assignment of participants to groups which vary only with respect to the experimental (independent) variable(s) (Campbell & Stanley, 1963).

courts and the clinics already in place), some key interest groups were skeptical about both the concept of community-based forensic groups and the nature of the training that community mental health clinicians would receive (see chapter 6). The pilot project was in part a compromise to placate those groups. Rather than embark with full force on a questionable course, the state would adopt a community-based model in a measured way with careful evaluation as an integral part of the program.

Second, despite the General Assembly's unequivocal finding of fact as to the workability of community-based forensic services, questions remained (e.g., the potential of a substantial net-widening effect) that could be answered only by systematically evaluating such a program. Third, the possibility of significant problems in implementing the program (e.g., judicial resistance) suggested the need to perform careful planning and evaluation of each step in full implementation. Such considerations seemed particularly significant because none of the previous studies had involved a program of the scope envisioned in Virginia.

Fourth, the disparities seemed justified in view of the need for research and the relatively unobjectionable nature of the disparities in conditions of evaluation.[34] Most of the remaining questions, which had substantial significance for policy, could not be easily studied in a simulation; a field test was necessary. All defendants, regardless of assignment to experimental condition, would be accorded an evaluation by qualified mental health professionals. The defendants in control jurisdictions would have the same conditions of evaluation as if the pilot project had not been initiated, and those in experimental jurisdictions could be expected to have evaluations of at least comparable quality. All defendants in a given jurisdiction would be accorded the same form of evaluation; thus, the disparities were between procedures across local *jurisdictions* rather than across individual defendants.[35]

Thus, the General Assembly's imprimatur for real-life study of community-

---

34. For discussion of factors to be used in assessing the ethics and constitutionality of disparate treatment resulting from proposed studies in the legal system, see Federal Judicial Center (1981).

The Supreme Court has never ruled directly on the constitutionality of disparity in treatment by the legal system on the basis of random assignment to experimental groups. However, in a review of disparity on the basis of offender characteristics in access to rehabilitative programs, the Supreme Court sanctioned broad legislative discretion in the allocation of limited resources in "essentially experimental program[s]" designed to deal with problems in "areas fraught with medical and scientific uncertainties." Marshall v. United States, 414 U.S. 417, 426–30 (1974).

35. In some sense, of course, the relevant jurisdiction is the state, not the local jurisdiction. Presumably, defendants charged with offenses on the basis of state law should be similarly treated throughout the state. Nonetheless, determination of where forensic evaluations were to be conducted had been a matter of trial judge discretion, although most chose to make referrals to the state forensic units. Therefore, the governing principles largely had been de facto rules in district and circuit courts. Assignment of *jurisdictions,* rather than *defendants,* to experimental conditions thus alleviates, but does not eliminate, concerns about equal protection of defendants.

based forensic services, even with an implicit foregone conclusion, gave a rare and, in our view, legitimate opportunity to conduct an experiment in the legal system. Besides providing a chance to study the efficacy of community-based forensic services in much more detail and with more rigorous control than in previous studies, the pilot project also offered an opportunity to learn more about the factors affecting interaction between the mental health and legal systems.

The Plan for This Book

Although both the Ohio and the Tennessee projects provided some basis for optimism about the feasibility of community-based forensic services, neither gave clear evidence of high quality and reduced costs. The remainder of this volume presents a comprehensive evaluation of the implementation of community-based forensic services in Virginia. Chapter 2 describes the initiation of community-based services in Virginia, the design of the evaluation research, and the effects of the program on admission rates and costs. Chapter 3 presents an evaluation of the level of specialized knowledge of clinicians in the program, and chapter 4 examines the quality of their reports. In chapter 5, data are presented on judges' attitudes toward the use of mental health professionals in various kinds of cases and on the form and frequency of involvement by community mental health professionals in the legal system. Chapter 6 describes the process of implementation of the program; anecdotes about problems encountered are presented, along with a list of dos and don'ts for the development of forensic services. The book concludes with policy recommendations in chapter 7, including appendixes of model authorizing legislation and court orders for forensic evaluation.

In general, the book addresses these questions in the following order: Do community-based forensic services really avoid some of the costs endemic to hospital-based services? Can community-based forensic clinicians develop sufficient expertise? Is that expertise reflected in their formal knowledge about relevant law and forensic clinical and research issues and the quality of their forensic evaluation reports? What can be said about the interaction between the courts and the mental health centers that would explain the success, or lack of success, in the program? Although the answers to these questions are most directly relevant to questions concerning the optimal organization of forensic services, they will also contribute, we think, to basic knowledge of the interaction between the mental health and legal systems.

Chapter 2

The Efficiency and Cost-Effectiveness of a Community-Based System of Forensic Evaluation

Evaluation of the Community-Based System in Virginia

THE RESEARCH DESIGN

Service needs and research considerations made it impossible to employ a true experimental design[1] in the evaluation of the Virginia community-based forensic service system. The closing of Southwestern State Hospital made the need for alternative forensic services especially serious for some regions of the state. Notably, the extreme southwestern part of Virginia is about three hundred miles from the remaining forensic unit at Central State Hospital in Petersburg, a formidable distance for transportation of defendants. Authorities were also anxious to include at least some of the state's largest cities in the pilot project, to reduce the already mounting pressure for admissions to Central State. The reality that only a few community mental health centers would be involved in the pilot project also made it unlikely that a representative group of them could be drawn by random selection.

For these reasons, we decided to adopt a quasi-experimental design (see Campbell & Stanley, 1963) that closely approximated a true experiment in the level of control of extraneous sources of variance. Specifically, a matching procedure was used to create a comparison group of community mental health catchment areas in which the status quo was preserved.[2] Six sites were selected as demonstration (experimental, *E*) clinics on the basis of geographic diversity (i.e., representation of each DMHMR region), service needs, and the

1. As used here, the term *experiment* does not refer to innovation per se. Rather, it is a technical term denoting research in which there is random assignment of participants to groups which vary only with respect to the experimental (independent) variable(s) (Campbell & Stanley, 1963).

2. We note with appreciation that, although we considered service needs in the initial design of the study, DMHMR was protective of that design once implemented. Thus, although some of the largest cities in the state (e.g., Norfolk)—and, therefore, some of the biggest contributors to the backlog of cases at Central State—were in the comparison group, DMHMR supported our refusal to include these jurisdictions in subsequent training programs until the completion of the pilot year in March 1982. However, service needs did require that the hospital-based outpatient system be implemented several months before the March 1982 date in those jurisdictions.

availability of psychiatrists. Specifically, *E* clinics were located in Alexandria, Charlottesville, Portsmouth, Radford, Richmond, and Roanoke. The entire catchment area for each *E* clinic was included in the project. Thus, in several instances, the center served a wide geographic area, including several court districts. In addition, the New River Valley Mental Health Center, located in Radford, took on responsibility as a regional center for evaluations of defendants located throughout southwest Virginia (west of the Roanoke Valley). However, for purposes of the study, only its own catchment area was included in analyses so the matching procedure was not distorted. In summary, though, the *E* jurisdictions represented a cross section of Virginia municipalities in terms of population density, socioeconomic variables, and access to professional resources.

The selection of the comparison (*C*) group, also composed of six community mental health centers, was a two-step matching procedure. The clinics in Virginia were divided into five groups on the basis of catchment area population. The six *E* clinics were then compared with clinics of similar catchment area size on the following variables which appeared to relate to clinics' willingness and capacity to perform forensic evaluations and to interact with the legal system effectively: clinic philosophy (i.e., nature of services offered, service goals, degree of outreach and community orientation); quality of clinic services (i.e., effectiveness and responsiveness to community needs); level of training and experience of staff; availability of outpatient mental health services in the private sector; size of staff. Ratings for similarity with the respective *E* clinics were made by DMHMR staff in the office of the assistant commissioner for community services who were familiar with the clinics across the state. The *C* clinics derived on this basis were located in Arlington, Chesapeake, Newport News, Norfolk, Petersburg, and Suffolk. The communities served by these community mental health centers appeared to be similarly representative of the state in terms of rural-suburban-urban and socioeconomic mix. Empirically, as we shall see, the success of the matching procedure was demonstrated by near-perfect matching of admissions to the inpatient forensic units in the two years prior to the onset of the pilot project.

In each of the *E* clinics, a forensic team averaging five clinicians, including at least one psychiatrist, was established. As described in more detail in chapter 6, these teams participated in at least eight days of training on relevant law, clinical technique, and research findings. The training program consisted of more than thirty hours of lecture and ten hours of supervised evaluation. The teams were given a manual of more than four hundred pages of xeroxed readings and outlines, and the formal didactic training was supplemented by occasional consultation and supervision by faculty from the Forensic Evaluation Training and Research Center.

For studies of effects of the pilot project on admission rates (this chapter) and report quality (chapter 4), direct comparisons of jurisdictions (E v. C) were undertaken. To test the effect of the project on the work of individual clinicians (i.e., their knowledge of forensic mental health, chapter 3; the quantity and nature of their interactions with officials in the legal system, chapter 5), clinicians in the E forensic teams were compared with several groups. One comparison group consisted of other (untrained) clinicians in the E clinics. Another comparison group consisted of all master's- and doctoral-level clinicians in the C clinics. Perhaps the most direct comparison was with a subgroup of staff from the C clinics who were identified by the clinic directors as being most likely to be included in a forensic team if the clinic were to establish one. This latter group is identified throughout this study as *director-designees*. Thus, care was taken to ensure that results were not biased by factors involved in the selection of the teams themselves.[3]

Finally, in addition to comparisons of E and C community clinics, E clinicians were compared with diplomates of the American Board of Forensic Psychology in their knowledge of the specialty (chapter 3) and with staff from Central State Hospital in the quality of their reports (chapter 4).

Because a primary impetus for the establishment of the community-based forensic evaluation system was the expectation that it would reduce admissions to the state hospitals, and thereby reduce evaluation costs as well as demands on inpatient services, we examined the program's effectiveness along these dimensions. Reductions in state hospital admissions for forensic evaluation are crucial to the success of a community-based system for a variety of reasons. Obviously, in implementing such a system, one hopes to find that the relevant legal professionals will increasingly use these community evaluation services and that this trend will be accompanied by a corresponding drop in the use of inpatient services. Rather than just widening the net, as it appears occurred with the Ohio program (see chapter 1), it was hoped that the Virginia program would effect a *transfer* in the site of forensic mental health services from the hospitals to the community clinics. This transfer was viewed as desirable for reasons (elaborated in chapter 1) relating to defendant rights, quality of services, and cost-effectiveness. In addition to these reasons, it was acknowl-

---

3. It was, of course, possible that the forensic teams included only the most skilled or most consultation-oriented clinicians in the E clinics. Conversely, if the forensic practice was perceived as undesirable or a drain on the resources of the mental health center, only the least competent clinicians might be assigned to this work.

edged that forensic units in the state hospital in Virginia were overcrowded, and defendants were often faced with substantial preadmission waiting periods as a result. This situation also reduced the quality of inpatient services, since the staff was overburdened. Further, the preadmission wait only served to extend the delay before trial for defendants referred for forensic evaluation.

In fact, the severe burden on Virginia's inpatient forensic services, combined with the state's optimism regarding the feasibility of outpatient forensic evaluations, led the Department of Mental Health and Mental Retardation also to develop a program of outpatient evaluations offered at the state hospitals. It was expected that the availability of such a program would increase the efficiency and cost-effectiveness of the services provided by the state hospital personnel. Whereas outpatient services within the defendant's jurisdiction were viewed as a preferred first-tier option, the DMHMR recognized that such services would not be available in all jurisdictions within Virginia for several years and considered outpatient hospital evaluations as a second-tier option, preferable to hospitalization.

In this chapter, we examine the data relating to the numbers of state hospital admissions for forensic evaluations from the experimental (E) and comparison (C) jurisdictions for four 1-year periods: (a) March 1, 1979, through February 29, 1980; (b) March 1, 1980, through February 28, 1981; (c) March 1, 1981, through February 28, 1982; and (d) March 1, 1982, through February 28, 1983. Corresponding data on frequencies of community-based and hospital-based outpatient evaluations also will be reported. Finally, costs estimated for those services will be discussed.

March 1, 1981, was the date of initiation of the community-based evaluation system in the E jurisdictions, and the subsequent twelve-month period was the pilot year of the program. During the March 1, 1982, through February 28, 1983, interval, the community-based program continued within the E jurisdictions. At varying points during the 1982–1983 year, the program also commenced in certain of the C jurisdictions, since, as reported below, data collected during the pilot year supported the continued expansion of the program into the rest of the state. In addition, the hospital-based outpatient program, available to some jurisdictions during the pilot year, was increasingly available during the 1982–1983 year. Ironically, the apparent success of the community-based program, as summarized in an interim six-month report to the DMHMR, may have inadvertently triggered the department's early initiation of the hospital-based outpatient program in the C jurisdictions late in the pilot year, despite the investigators' requests that confounding influences, such as availability of a *third* variety of forensic services in the jurisdictions under study, not occur during that evaluation year.

The response of DMHMR to the initial, apparent success of the pilot program is representative of a more general phenomenon. As an experimental program of intervention appears to be successful, pressure may be exerted to abandon formal evaluation and its concomitant controls to facilitate full-scale implementation. A tension often exists between the requirements of scientific rigor in program evaluation and service needs, necessitating a continuing balance and cooperative negotiation among participants throughout the evaluation process.

Admissions to State Hospitals for Forensic Evaluations

METHOD

Frequencies of state hospital admissions for forensic evaluations were derived from two sources: the DMHMR's automated Management Information System (MIS) and manual tabulations by state hospital personnel. In Virginia, all persons admitted to state hospitals are assigned a legal status code which reflects the reason for their admission through reference to the statutory authority for that admission. Thus, persons admitted for forensic evaluation were typically admitted under the statutory authority of Virginia Code Section 19.2-169,[4] and were assigned the appropriate legal status code, which is subsequently entered into the MIS. We retrieved such data for the time intervals of interest for each of the E and C jurisdictions.[5]

We learned, however, that the director of forensic services in a major state hospital had recently begun encouraging statewide use of a different coding procedure with certain forensic admissions. Apparently a small proportion of defendants admitted for forensic evaluation also required intensive treatment

---

4. Va. Code § 19.2-169 (Supp. 1982).

5. This automated data base provided numbers of admissions for forensic evaluations according to the jurisdiction of each defendant's legal residence. Our primary interest, however, was not in the jurisdictions of defendants' legal residence, but in the jurisdictions in which the defendants were alleged to have committed the crimes and were facing legal proceedings, and therefore, from which they were admitted. We expected that the large percentage of crimes would be committed in the same jurisdictions in which offenders resided. We had available to us manual data from the primary forensic unit in Virginia, which identified each defendant's residential as well as admitting jurisdiction. Our calculations ($N = 110$) revealed that most defendants face legal proceedings in, and are thus admitted from, the same jurisdiction where they reside. Further, when the jurisdictions differ, no systematic pattern was observed. It appeared that the small deviations revealed were roughly similar in experimental and comparison jurisdictions. Further, the number of defendants *not* residing in a particular jurisdiction where they were facing charges was approximately similar to the number of defendants residing in a particular jurisdiction but facing legal charges elsewhere, thus virtually "cancelling out" numerical discrepancies.

and were viewed as being seriously enough disturbed to meet the state's civil commitment criteria. For those individuals, it was recommended that they be admitted under the statutory authority of the civil commitment statute,[6] and that forensic evaluations be performed during their course of treatment. It appeared that this practice, which had not reached the status of a formal policy, was implemented somewhat unsystematically throughout the state hospital system. The MIS was unable to process multiple concurrent reasons for admission (i.e., legal status codes). Thus, it was not possible for the automated system to record these individuals as users of both forensic evaluation *and* mental health treatment resources.[7] Therefore, data relating to these individuals were tabulated manually. Fortunately, record keeping at the state hospitals was sufficiently organized that these data were accessible for past as well as current years.

As noted above, admissions data were collected for each of the six *E* and six *C* jurisdictions during two preprogram years (1979–1980 and 1980–1981), the pilot year (1981–1982), and the subsequent year (1982–1983).

RESULTS

The frequency of state hospital admissions for forensic evaluation for the two years prior to the initiation of the community-based program was compared with that of the pilot year of the program and the year after. The frequencies are reported in Table 1 and are depicted graphically in Figure 1. The data indicate that in the two years prior to the onset of the new program, the total number of admissions to hospitals for forensic evaluation from both the *E* and *C* groups remained relatively constant. The data also reveal that the total number of hospital admissions for forensic evaluation from the *E* versus *C* group during the preprogram years were remarkably similar (providing further evidence for the validity of the matching of the *E* and *C* clinics). Most important, however, Table 1 reveals that during the pilot year of the community-based program, the frequency of admissions to state hospitals for forensic evaluations dropped 46.38 percent in the *E* jurisdictions, when compared with the mean of the two previous years; whereas the frequency of admissions in the *C* areas remained constant. A chi-square test comparing the mean of the two previous years with the frequency of the pilot year in the *E* versus *C* jurisdictions was significant at the .001 level, χ^2 (1, $N = 730$) = 12.26.

6. Va. Code §§ 37.1-67.1 to 37.1-67.3 (Supp. 1982).

7. In the course of the evaluation research described in this book, we began to work with DMHMR and the Supreme Court of Virginia to facilitate revisions in the capacities of the automated data systems to process valid forensic mental health data. The collaboration between the Institute of Law, Psychiatry and Public Policy and the state on these projects continues. Unfortunately, budgetary problems have slowed the state's progress with their plans for revising their automated hospital-based system and for developing a new automated system for community mental health centers.

Table 1: Hospital Admissions for Forensic Evaluation
in the Experimental and Comparison Jurisdictions

Experimental Jurisdictions	1979–80	1980–81	1981–82	1982–83
A	20	23	23	13
B	22	13	3	6
C	27	23	13	12
D	19	10	2	3
E	59	86	59	43
F	67	45	11	13
Total Admissions	214	200	111	90

Comparison Jurisdictions	1979–80	1980–81	1981–82	1982–83
G	17	18	28	16
H	11	14	11	7
I	59	55	31	26
J	72	57	58	17
K	51	34	52	21
L	19	23	17	6
Total Admissions	229	201	197	93

Note: Hospital admissions include admissions to all hospitals under Section 19.2-169 and admissions of persons who received forensic evaluations while hospitalized under section 37.1-67.1. The total number of persons who received forensic evaluation while hospitalized under 37.1-67.1 was eight in the experimental jurisdictions and four in the comparison jurisdictions.

We continued to track the frequency of admissions during the 1982–1983 year to ascertain whether the observed changes would be maintained. As noted in Table 1, the reduction in admissions was maintained and may have continued to drop slightly in the E jurisdictions during the 1982–1983 year to a level that was 56.52 percent lower than in the preprogram years. However, because the pilot year of the project ended on February 28, 1982, community-based and hospital-based outpatient services became available within several of the C jurisdictions, invalidating further statistical comparisons between the E and C groups. Thus it is unclear whether the apparent further reduction in hospital admissions in the E jurisdictions in 1982 and 1983 is an index of a trend toward increasing reductions or reflects nonsystematic yearly fluctuations in admissions rates. As also indicated in Table 1, during the 1982–1983 year, admis-

30

Figure 1: Admissions to Virginia State Hospitals for Forensic Evaluations in the Experimental and Comparison Jurisdictions (March 1, 1979–February 28, 1983)

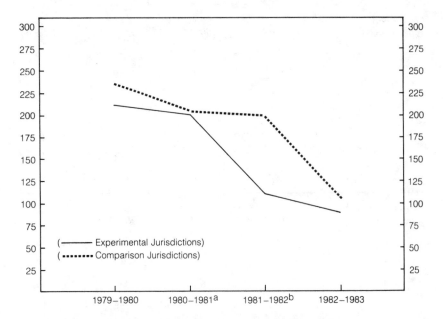

aMarch 1, 1981, was the onset of the pilot project in the experimental jurisdictions.
bDuring 1981–1982, community- and hospital-based forensic evaluation services became available in the comparison jurisdictions.

sions for forensic evaluations in the C jurisdictions dropped to ninety-three, or 55.5 percent of the mean for the previous three years.

Examination of the reductions in hospital admissions within the particular E jurisdictions reveals much variability. Admissions in jurisdictions B, D, and F dropped by over 80 percent when the pilot-year frequencies are compared with the mean of the two preprogram years. Admissions in jurisdiction C were reduced by about 50 percent; whereas admissions in jurisdictions A and E appeared not to change.

DISCUSSION

The reduction in admissions in the E jurisdictions during the pilot year of the program suggests that the availability of community-based forensic evaluation services in those jurisdictions had a significant impact on the rate of hospital admissions for forensic evaluation. In addition, these reductions in admissions were maintained during the subsequent year. Further analysis of the admissions data leads us to speculate that it might be possible for this type of program to reduce hospital admissions even more. The pattern of changes within the particular *E* jurisdictions corresponded to our expectations, given how well we perceived the implementation of the program to be progressing within these jurisdictions. The relevant legal professionals (judges and attorneys) had been contacted and were receptive in jurisdictions B, D, and F, and the forensic teams at the community mental health centers within those jurisdictions appeared to be competent and motivated to participate. The result was a reduction in admissions for forensic evaluations of over 80 percent. We expect that this reduction is attributable to the successful implementation and smooth operation of the community-based program within those jurisdictions.

We attributed the *lack* of success in jurisdiction A to an ongoing problem with two district court judges. These judges, who were responsible for the large percentage of forensic evaluation referrals in that jurisdiction, were unwilling to work with the community mental health center, for reasons which were never completely clear but may have been related to personalities or previous experiences with mental health professionals. The mental health professionals in that jurisdiction performed exceedingly well on the competence measures described in chapters 3 and 4, which suggests that their demonstrated level of expertise was not the source of the problem. During the subsequent year, 1982 to 1983, efforts were made by the faculty at the Institute of Law, Psychiatry and Public Policy to work with these judges and to address their concerns. Those efforts may be partly reflected in the reduction in admissions for jurisdiction A in the second postprogram year.

Jurisdiction E, a relatively large urban area, presented a somewhat different and more challenging problem. Approximately fourteen judges were responsible for referrals for forensic evaluation (and correspondingly high numbers of prosecuting and defense attorneys) within that jurisdiction. Prior to the pilot program, and throughout the pilot year, the Institute of Law, Psychiatry and Public Policy was not able to secure meetings with all of the legal professionals involved. Many meetings with judges to describe the program were scheduled and held, yet attendance was often poor, and success was not easily forthcoming. Despite continued efforts in the postpilot year, admissions appeared to drop only slightly over previous years, although the efforts may gradually have had an impact. Further, there appeared to be some skepticism about the qualifications of the community mental health staff among these legal professionals, many of whom had existing working relationships with the staff at the primary inpatient forensic facility and with private clinicians. Finally, the proximity of this jurisdiction to the state hospital and therefore accessibility to that facility may also have mitigated against an easy transition. It is not clear that all large urban centers will present such difficulties, however. Jurisdiction J, an urban area, began participating in the program early in the second program year, and admissions appeared to drop substantially during that year.

Finally, there were no problems with legal professionals in jurisdiction C, where admissions dropped about 50 percent, but a key mental health professional in the community mental health center resisted the program and apparently encouraged legal professionals to refer cases to the state hospital rather than to the clinic.

We might speculate that the 80 percent reduction in admissions may be close to the highest level possible. Some defendants will always be referred for forensic evaluation because they require inpatient hospitalization for dangerous behavior not easily contained in jail, a concurrent need for inpatient treatment, or an actual need for daily observation and extended evaluation. Although we cannot estimate what proportion of referrals falls into these categories, our experience with jurisdictions B, D, and F would suggest that it is certainly not greater than 20 percent of those persons who otherwise might have been hospitalized, and may even be lower. Interestingly, our findings are consistent with those in the Tennessee program (Laben & Spencer, 1976), in which it was reported that approximately 20 percent of referrals to community centers are eventually hospitalized for further evaluation (M. Whitlock, personal communication).

A rather impressive drop in admissions also occurred in the C jurisdictions during the first postpilot year. During that year, staff in four of the C clinics received forensic training. In addition, the outpatient hospital-based evaluation system became available. This reduction in admissions will be discussed in greater detail in the next section.

In summary, therefore, it appears that the availability of community-based forensic evaluation services can lead to substantial stable reductions in hospital admissions for such evaluations. However, the success of this type of program in reducing admissions appears to be directly related to the willingness of both the mental health and legal professionals involved to collaborate with one another. Lack of information, negative attitudes, and biases all might contribute to a lower rate of success of the program in a particular jurisdiction. Such findings strongly underscore the importance of adequate training and education for all persons involved in the proposed collaboration and of identifying and addressing more general as well as idiosyncratic concerns about the program.

Use of the Community-Based Forensic Evaluation Services

The substantial reductions in hospital admissions in the E jurisdictions during the pilot year strongly suggest that the community-based program was achieving its first objective. We then examined frequencies of referrals for community-based and hospital-based outpatient evaluations in the E and C jurisdictions for the four-year period we were studying. Clearly, the possible net-widening effect of the availability of a high-quality, convenient, and lower-cost service in the community required further evaluation.

METHOD

Under the DMHMR Management Information System, only inpatient hospital data is coded. Thus, frequencies of community-based and hospital-based out-patient evaluations were tabulated by the personnel at each facility. Fortunately, the state hospitals, having performed forensic evaluations for many years, kept records of all such evaluations performed on both an inpatient and outpatient basis. Therefore, we were able to obtain data regarding outpatient evaluations from the hospitals retrospectively for both of the preprogram years as well as for the pilot and subsequent years. By contrast, prior to the onset of the pilot program, the community mental health centers did not record such data. Although the professionals reported having performed occasional forensic evaluations prior to the onset of the program, no data regarding such evaluations were available. The court system also did not record such information. The E clinic personnel did, however, tabulate numbers of evaluations performed during the 1981–1982 and 1982–1983 years. C clinic staff collected such data during the pilot year only.

One additional complicating factor is that prior to the onset of the pilot program, forensic evaluations were conducted with some regularity by jail physicians and private mental health professionals. Again, no data were available regarding the frequencies of these evaluations in current or prior years. Therefore, we attempted to estimate the number of evaluations performed during these years through figures obtained from the Supreme Court of Virginia. These figures do not report numbers of forensic evaluations ordered. Rather, they indicate the total amount of fees paid for forensic evaluations within each jurisdiction over a given period of time. It also was not possible to ascertain from these records who was the recipient of such payments. Given that only aggregate sums expended for forensic evaluations were available, we estimated the number of evaluations performed in each jurisdiction by dividing the aggregate by the cost of the average forensic evaluation conducted by jail physicians, private mental health professionals, and community centers. The average cost of each evaluation was estimated at $75 by Supreme Court data systems personnel.[8] Such estimates were only possible during the preprogram years within

---

8. This average figure represents a range of approximately $50 to $300. Most evaluations performed by jail physicians of competency to stand trial cost approximately $50 and probably made up the overwhelming proportion of payments. More comprehensive evaluations, which were less frequent, were increasingly expensive.

the E jurisdictions, because the fee structure changed with the onset of the pilot year.

We will report the total numbers of forensic evaluations performed in the E and C jurisdictions, to the best estimate of the investigators, during the four-year period. The data estimated for the community-based evaluations are listed in parentheses (in Table 2) to emphasize their approximate nature, as are the numbers of evaluations which are derived, in part, from totals of community-based evaluations. The estimates for the 1979–1980 and 1980–1981 years within the E jurisdictions, and for these two years plus the pilot year for the C jurisdictions, were derived from the Supreme Court aggregate fiscal data. The data for the pilot year and subsequent year, 1981–1982 and 1982–1983, for the E jurisdictions were tabulated by the community mental health clinic personnel. These latter figures do not include numbers of evaluations conducted by private mental health professionals or jail physicians because changes in fee structures at the onset of the program prevented further estimation of such data, which were not available elsewhere. However, reports from staff in the E clinics and from the courts suggest that a small number of such evaluations *were* conducted in three areas which happened to be those with the least reduction in hospital admissions. Thus, the figures we report for community-based evaluations for the latter two years may be a slight underestimation for jurisdictions A, C, and E, and the implications will be discussed.

RESULTS

Table 2 presents our best estimates of the total number of evaluations performed in the E and C jurisdictions during the four 1-year periods studied. It appears that during the two preprogram years, the numbers of community-based evaluations remained relatively constant in both groups. During the 1981–1982 year, when the community-based forensic program was implemented in the E jurisdictions, community forensic evaluations increased about 42 percent from the mean of the two previous years in those jurisdictions; whereas it continued to remain relatively stable in the C areas. Given that the 1981–1982 total for the E jurisdictions probably is a slight underestimate because it does not take into account evaluations conducted by jail physicians or private mental health professionals, we might estimate a slightly higher increase in the number of community evaluations during this year. During the next year, community-based evaluations in the E jurisdictions increased to a total which was 66.34 percent greater than the estimates of preprogram years.

Table 2 reveals that although the use of the hospital-based outpatient program is almost negligible in the E jurisdictions, it is substantial in the C jurisdictions. During the 1982–1983 year, hospital admissions dropped in the C jurisdictions by 55.5 percent of the mean for the previous three years, while use of the hospital outpatient system appeared to increase markedly. No data were available on numbers of community-based evaluations in the *C* jurisdictions during that year, and estimates could not be computed from Supreme Court records because the evaluation systems shifted from hospital-based to community-based at various points during the year for different jurisdictions, thus changing fee schedules.

An examination of the estimates for the total numbers of forensic evaluations performed in the *E* jurisdictions over the four-year period indicates that during the two preprogram years and the pilot year, the level of total evaluations remained relatively constant. During the first postpilot year, however, the total number of evaluations appeared to increase about 10 percent over previous years.

DISCUSSION

These data strongly suggest that the onset of the formal state-run community-based system of forensic evaluations in the *E* clinics was not accompanied by a substantial increase in the total number of evaluations conducted. It appears that during the second year the program was operating in the *E* clinics, 1982 to 1983, community-based services were increasingly used, and such use was not always accompanied by a correspondingly large drop in hospital admissions. Such a finding suggests that the existence of the community services may have slightly increased the number of evaluations requested. Persons who might not have been referred for evaluation in previous years might now be receiving community evaluations. As noted, these data probably are a slight underestimate because we were unable to obtain data relating to the small numbers of jail and private evaluations. However, the 10 percent, or slightly greater, increase in total evaluations during the 1982–1983 year over previous years is sufficiently small enough to allay undue concern about inappropriate use of community services. Cost data presented below support this conclusion. In fact, one might interpret this increase as a positive finding. This 10 percent might represent persons who needed forensic evaluations but did not receive them under the previous system.

During the 1982–1983 year, staff in four of the six *C* clinics received forensic training and began performing outpatient forensic evaluations. Clinic I became available for outpatient evaluations in June 1982, clinic J in April 1982, clinic K in January 1982, and clinic L in July 1982. And, as noted above, during this year, admissions for forensic evaluations dropped by 55.5 percent. That drop was probably associated with the availability of *both* the hospital-based and community-based outpatient services. (It is not possible to tease out the relative

Table 2: Total Forensic Evaluations in the Experimental and Comparison Jurisdictions (March 1, 1979–February 28, 1983)

Experimental Jurisdictions	Hospital Admissions[a]				Community-Based Evaluations			
	79–80	80–81	81–82	82–83	79–80[b]	80–81[b]	81–82[c]	82–83[c]
A	20	23	23	13	(47)	(34)	(41)	(58)
B	22	13	3	6	(3)	(0)	(41)	(25)
C	27	23	13	12	(40)	(21)	(28)	(16)
D	19	10	2	3	(1)	(1)	(10)	(40)
E	59	86	59	43	(37)	(108)	(111)	(127)
F	67	45	11	13	(37)	(48)	(60)	(75)
Total	214	200	111	90	(198)	(212)	(291)	(341)

Comparison Jurisdictions	79–80	80–81	81–82	82–83	79–80[b]	80–81[b]	81–82[g]	82–83[h]
G	17	18	28	16	(122)	(117)	(120)	
H	11	14	11	7	(29)	(14)	(37)	
I[f]	59	55	31	26	(1)	(0)	(0)	
J[f]	72	57	58	17	(58)	(45)	(33)	
K[f]	51	34	52	21	(0)	(0)	(0)	
L[f]	19	23	17	6	(5)	(0)	(0)	
Total	229	201	197	93	(215)	(176)	(190)	

a. Hospital admissions include admissions to all hospitals under Virginia Code Section 19.2-169 and admissions of persons who received forensic evaluations while hospitalized under Virginia Code Section 37.1-67.1. The total number of persons who received forensic evaluations while hospitalized under 37.1-67.1 was eight in the experimental jurisdictions and four in the comparison jurisdictions.

b. These figures were estimated from data provided by the Supreme Court of Virginia on court expenditures for community-based forensic evaluations. The recipients of such payment include community mental health centers, jail physicians, and private mental health practitioners. These figures are in parentheses to emphasize their approximate nature.

c. These figures include all forensic evaluations performed by the community mental health centers in the experimental jurisdictions as reported by the centers. These figures are in parentheses to indicate that they do not include frequencies of community evaluations performed by jail and private clinicians and are therefore slight underestimates.

impact of each during this transition year.) Where community-based services had been available and established in the E jurisdictions, there does not appear to be a similarly strong preference for the newly available hospital outpatient services. It is possible therefore that as community-based forensic evaluation services become better established and as implementation problems are worked out within the C jurisdictions, use of the community mental health center

Hospital Outpatient Evaluations[d]				Total Evaluations[e]			
79–80	80–81	81–82	82–83	79–80	80–81	81–82	82–83
0	0	0	5	(67)	(67)	(64)	(76)
0	1	1	0	(25)	(14)	(45)	(31)
0	1	0	6	(67)	(45)	(41)	(34)
0	2	0	0	(20)	(13)	(12)	(43)
1	3	11	8	(130)	(197)	(181)	(178)
0	0	2	6	(104)	(93)	(73)	(94)
1	7	14	25	(413)	(419)	(416)	(456)

79–80	80–81	81–82	82–83	79–80	80–81	81–82	82–83[h]
0	0	0	3	(139)	(135)	(148)	
0	0	2	4	(40)	(28)	(50)	
0	0	13	45	(60)	(55)	(44)	
3	5	14	16	(133)	(107)	(105)	
12	5	12	22	(63)	(39)	(64)	
0	0	4	8	(24)	(23)	(21)	
15	10	45	99	(459)	(387)	(432)	

d. These data were provided by the four major state hospitals.

e. These data are in parentheses to indicate their approximate nature (see notes b and c).

f. These four jurisdictions received forensic training and began performing outpatient forensic evaluations during the 1982–1983 year. They were trained at different points during that year: J (April 1982); I (June 1982); L (July 1982); K (January 1983).

g. Of the 190 community-based forensic evaluations in the comparison jurisdictions during the 1981–1982 year, 13 were performed by the community mental health centers. The remaining 177 evaluations were conducted by jail physicians or private practitioners.

h. The total number of evaluations for the comparison jurisdictions for 1982–1983 is not directly comparable to the totals of previous years because the evaluation systems (hospital-based versus community-based) shifted at various points during the year for different jurisdictions. Thus no figures were tabulated for this transition year, and no totals were tabulated for total evaluations.

services will increase, and use of the somewhat less convenient and less accessible hospital-based outpatient services will decrease.

Overall, however, it does appear that the introduction of the community-based system has led to a *redistribution* of forensic evaluations from the hospital inpatient units to the community mental health centers with minimal net increases in total evaluations. Further, evaluations previously performed within the community by jail physicians or private mental health professionals appear also to have shifted to the community mental health centers. These latter shifts are viewed positively because jail physicians in Virginia are not regarded as having the expertise necessary to perform competent forensic mental health evaluations and because payment to private mental health professionals diverts funds from public agencies. Thus, the benefits of such a redistribution may be felt both in quality of services and in financial advantages.

Where available, forensic evaluation services by community mental health professionals seem to be preferred over hospital-based outpatient services. Yet, when the former are either unavailable or not well established, hospital-based outpatient services may be used and may lead to substantial reductions in hospital admissions.

The Cost-Effectiveness of the Community-Based System

Although policymakers in Virginia were concerned about the benefits of a community-based system for defendant civil rights, quality of services, and lessening the burden on the overtaxed hospital system, a primary motivation to pursue the community-based program was its expected cost savings. We therefore estimated the relative cost of an inpatient versus community-based forensic evaluation system.

METHOD

We estimated expenditures for each type of service required for the community-based, inpatient, and hospital outpatient evaluations and computed an approximate cost comparison in a manner similar to that employed by Laben et al. (1977). We found that the cost of outpatient services rose in 1981–1982, and the cost of inpatient services rose between the pilot year and the next year; thus we calculated varying costs for those two years accordingly.

To approximate the cost of hospitalization for forensic evaluation in 1981 to 1982 and in previous years, we assumed a thirty-day hospitalization, because previous data obtained by the institute both in 1977 (McCall, 1979) and in 1981 (Slobogin, Melton, & Showalter, 1984) suggested that estimate. The per diem cost of inpatient hospitalization was estimated at $85 by the assistant director for administration at the state hospital with the largest forensic unit. This per diem cost rose to $110 for the 1982–1983 year and subsequent years. One sheriff's deputy would accompany all defendants to the state hospitals and would typically require lunch (estimated by the sheriff's department at $5). The cost of transportation between the local jail and the state hospital was estimated at $40 (twenty cents per mile) with an average transport of two hundred miles round trip (although the typical round trip may range from ten miles to six hundred miles). Because the deputies would make one round trip to deliver the defendant and a second round trip approximately thirty days later to retrieve the defendant, these costs (transport and lunch) were doubled. No salaries or overtime were included in these computations, since deputies are paid a flat rate, regardless of duties performed or actual hours logged. It was also typical for defendants to average ten days in jail between their return from the hospital and their first court appearance, and a cost of $15 per day was derived as an average of the rates in the various jails serving the E jurisdictions. During the 1981– 1982 year, and for previous years, these figures led to an estimated cost for each inpatient evaluation of $2,790. During the 1982–1983 year, because of the rising cost of hospitalization, the estimated cost for each inpatient evaluation was $3,540.

To compute the cost of community evaluations, we assumed the average of $75 per evaluation in the preprogram years, since this estimate had been provided by the personnel at the Supreme Court of Virginia. In the pilot year, and in subsequent years, the average fee for a community-based evaluation was estimated to be $150, based on standardized rates implemented with the onset of the new program. Defendants were expected to stay approximately twenty days in jail, according to several Virginia district court judges, who indicated that when defendants who are referred for evaluations are not hospitalized, the time period between arrest and first court appearance is cut approximately in half. The daily expense of jail was estimated at $15. In most instances, community mental health center staff evaluated the defendants in the jail. In others, however, deputies transported the defendants to the mental health centers for evaluation. In either case, we estimated that the round-trip mileage would be approximately ten miles at twenty cents per mile (i.e., $5). Thus the cost for each evaluation during the prepilot years would be approximately $380, and the cost of each evaluation during the pilot year and subsequent year was estimated at $455.

To calculate the cost of hospital outpatient evaluations, we assumed an average cost of $151 for professional and clerical services provided by state hospital personnel, as estimated by the administrator of the forensic unit at the primary state hospital performing forensic evaluations. The average jail stay of twenty days at $15 per day (i.e., $300) was calculated, as was the average cost per round trip of one hundred fifty miles at twenty cents per mile, plus the $5 cost of the deputy's lunch. The approximate cost of each outpatient hospital evaluation was $486.

Table 3: Estimated Costs for Forensic Evaluations
in Experimental Jurisdictions (March 1, 1979 through February 28, 1973)

	1979–1980		1980–1981	
	Number of Evaluations	Estimated Cost	Number of Evaluations	Estimated Cost
Hospital admissions[a]	214	$597,060[d]	200	$588,000[d]
Hospital outpatient evaluations[b]	1	$486	7	$3,402
Community-based evaluations[c]	198	$75,240	212	$80,560
Totals	413	$672,786[d]	419	$641,962[d]

a. At estimated average cost of $2,790 each in 1979–1980, 1980–1981, and 1981–1982, and cost of $3,540 each in 1982–1983.

b. At estimated average cost of $486 each.

c. At estimated average cost of $380 each in 1979–1980 and 1980–1981, and $455 each in 1981–1982 and 1982–1983.

RESULTS

Using these figures, we calculated the estimated expenses of providing forensic evaluation services during the two preprogram years, the pilot year, and the subsequent year and report those estimates in Table 3. The data indicate that the overall estimated cost to the state of providing forensic evaluations within the *E* jurisdictions dropped from a preprogram mean of $657,374 to $485,905 in 1982 to 1983, saving $171,469, or 26.08 percent. Since the per diem expense for hospitalization at the forensic units rose from $85 in previous years to $110 in 1982 to 1983, the reported saving probably is an underestimate. If inpatient evaluations had remained at their preprogram mean of 207 per year, the cost of inpatient evaluations in the *E* jurisdictions that year would have been approximately $732,780, bringing the expected total cost of forensic evaluations to an estimated $812,624. Compared with the 1982–1983 figures, these totals suggest an estimated saving of $326,719, or 40.21 percent within those jurisdictions.

DISCUSSION

The postprogram years saw a slight increase (approximately 10 percent) in the total number of forensic evaluations performed within the *E* jurisdictions and a two-fold increase in the cost of such evaluations (caused primarily by the higher fee structure instituted as part of the new program to provide incentives for community mental health professionals to participate in the program). Yet, despite these increases, the estimated cost savings within the *E* jurisdictions was

1981–1982		1982–1983	
Number of Evaluations	Estimated Cost	Number of Evaluations	Estimated Cost
111	$309,690[d]	90	$318,600[d]
14	$6,804	25	$12,150
291	$132,405	341	$155,155
416	$448,899[d]	456	$485,905[d]

d. Since the per diem cost for inpatient service increased from $85 to $110 in 1982–1983, the figures listed here for inpatient evaluations are not directly comparable across years. If the numbers of inpatient versus outpatient evaluations had remained at their preprogram rate of approximately 207 per year (mean of 1979–1980 and 1980–1981 rates), the cost of inpatient evaluations at the new per diem cost would have been $732,780, bringing the mean cost of total evaluations to approximately $812,624, as compared with the 1982–1983 total estimated cost of $485,905.

$326,719, or approximately 40 percent. This calculation assumes that the number of inpatient evaluations would have remained relatively stable at preprogram levels over the four-year period had the community-based system not been implemented. If one considers that there are forty Community Services Boards in Virginia and that the E jurisdictions tap into only six, one might predict that the potential cost savings to the state would be great. It is expected that cost savings might be even greater over time, if implementation difficulties, such as those identified for jurisdictions A, C, and E, were ameliorated, because cost savings in the three more successful jurisdictions are estimated at approximately 55 percent.

Two notes of caution are warranted at this juncture. First, as noted above, we probably are underestimating slightly the total number of outpatient evaluations performed in the postprogram years. Second, these cost estimates do not include the start-up expenses associated with this type of program. The cost of training the community mental health professionals and of educating legal professionals is assumed by the state. Again, while this raises the estimated cost, we expect that dramatic overall cost savings would still be found.

However, as noted earlier in this chapter, and in chapter 1, expected cost savings alone are only one of several reasons why it might be beneficial for a state to institute a community-based system of forensic evaluations. In Virginia, it was of great importance that the excessive demand (which revealed itself in overcrowding and preadmission waiting periods) be lifted from the state hospital forensic units—a goal that appears to have been accomplished in the E jurisdictions increasing the efficiency of the forensic system. In addition, it appears that the program may have additional positive, nonspecific effects on the efficiency and quality of other public services. For example, sheriff's deputies were typically removed from other law enforcement duties to accompany defendants to state hospitals. Most community mental health center staff perform forensic evaluations in the jails, alleviating this burden on the sheriff's department. In addition, one sheriff reported that the onset of the program in his jurisdiction had a positive impact not only on the capacity of the sheriff's department to perform law enforcement duties, but on the morale of the deputies. Assuming that the findings regarding quality of services presented in the following chapters are convincing, the community-based system will have succeeded in accomplishing multiple goals simultaneously: increasing the efficiency of the system, improving the quality of services, and reducing overall cost.

Chapter 3

Knowledge of Forensic Issues among
Community Mental Health Professionals

The preceding chapter provides strong support for the notion that a community-based system of forensic services results in substantial fiscal savings while reducing unnecessary intrusions into defendants' interests in bail and a speedy trial. The state and the defendant would not be well served, however, if the *quality* of the outpatient evaluation was significantly poorer than that obtained as an inpatient. Therefore, as part of the evaluation of the Virginia program, it was also important to assess the quality of the forensic evaluations.

One component of quality of forensic evaluations is the level of expertise of the evaluator. In most jurisdictions, the test of whether the opinion of a mental health professional is admissible as evidence is whether the opinion is based on *specialized knowledge* that will *assist the trier of fact* (i.e., the judge or the jury) in determination of a *relevant* issue.[1] Therefore, we decided to assess the relative level of the forensic teams' knowledge of law, research, and clinical issues relevant to criminal and juvenile mental health practice. Did the forensic clinicians attain a corpus of knowledge similar to board-certified forensic clinicians? Was the forensic clinicians' level of knowledge "specialized" in comparison to that of general mental health professionals and trial judges?

The answer to the latter question is important not only in the context of the evaluation of the Virginia pilot project. It also has considerable significance in an ongoing controversy in mental health law concerning the question of which, if any, opinions of mental health professionals should be admissible. The gadfly in this debate has been Morse (1978, 1982a, 1982b) who has argued articulately that mental health professionals should be barred from providing any opinions about a defendant's mental state in testimony. Rather, he would limit mental health professionals' role to giving behavioral descriptions and, when available and relevant, hard actuarial data. Morse rests his conclusions on several arguments: (a) cases in mental health law generally involve moral and legal decisions, not scientific determinations; (b) the necessary inferences about human behavior are commonsense judgments within the purview of the fact

1. Fed. R. Evid. 702.

finder; (c) the scientific basis of mental health professionals' opinions is so limited that it lacks substantial probative value.

In commentary on Morse's position, we and our colleagues (Bonnie & Slobogin, 1980; Melton et al., in press, chap. 1) fully concur that mental health professionals should be neither permitted nor cajoled into giving ultimate legal opinions (e.g., whether a defendant was insane at the time of the offense, whether a respondent is so dangerous as to warrant civil commitment). Scholarly commentary (see, e.g., ABA, 1983; American Psychiatric Association, 1982; Bazelon, 1982; Comment, 1979; Task Force on the Role of Psychology in the Criminal Justice System, 1978) is nearly unanimous that the ultimate issue involves legal and moral line-drawing, about which mental health professionals have no particular expertise. Thus, despite the favor with which many legal practitioners regard de facto abdication of decisions in mental health law to clinicians (Poythress, 1978, 1982a, 1982b, 1983), ultimate-issue opinions of mental health professionals should be inadmissible.

We part company, however, with Morse in his argument that mental health professionals' formulations and diagnoses should also be inadmissible. At root, this disagreement turns on differences in perception of the level of specialized knowledge possessed by mental health experts. In our view, a relevant body of psychological knowledge often exists outside the ken of the fact finder and is sufficiently probative to outweigh its prejudicial value. In short, we have argued that mental health professionals' impressions and formulations often *do* assist fact finders in decision making. We have also contended, however, that credentials as a mental health professional (or as a professional in a particular mental health discipline) are insufficient to establish a proffered expert's ability to assist the fact finder. Rather, the question should be whether the clinician possesses specialized knowledge of the particular issue at hand (e.g., the prediction of dangerousness).

Development of a Test of Forensic Knowledge

To be competent in forensic evaluation, mental health professionals need three general types of knowledge in addition to basic competence as a clinician. First, they need to be knowledgeable about relevant law, with respect both to the legal questions which evaluations must address (e.g., the elements of competency to stand trial) and to law governing forensic practice (e.g., fifth amendment issues in forensic evaluation, standards for admission of expert testimony). In addition, they need to be sufficiently knowledgeable about the legal system itself to be comfortable and adroit in communicating their opinions. Finally, forensic clinicians should be conversant with general legal concepts, including prevailing federal law, and the law and legal system in their state. Second, forensic evaluators need to be experts concerning research relevant to particular psychological questions (e.g., factors affecting competency to waive *Miranda* rights) and particular psychological conditions that are frequently the subject of forensic consultation (e.g., factors affecting amenability to treatment of sex offenders). Third, forensic mental health professionals need to be knowledgeable about clinical issues in forensic practice (e.g., means of information gathering).

We constructed an eighty-item multiple-choice test to measure knowledge in each of these areas. Specifically, sixteen items were generated with respect to each of the common domains of criminal and juvenile mental health law: general forensic issues, competency to stand trial, mental state at the time of the offense, sentencing, and juvenile law. For each of these domains, there were four-item cells on national law, Virginia law, research, and clinical issues. Thus, there were, in effect, nine subtest scores and an overall test score to be obtained.

In generating the items, care was taken to ensure content validity (i.e., to ensure that the items were representative of the universe of possible items in each cell). A pool of items was generated by the psychiatrists, psychologists, and lawyers who were professors or fellows in the Institute of Law, Psychiatry and Public Policy at the time (1981). Two of us (Melton and Slobogin) then edited these items into drafts of the test. Each draft was presented to the institute faculty and fellows for critique of both the exam as a whole and individual items with respect to representativeness, comprehensiveness, accuracy, and clarity. Rewriting, addition, and deletion of items followed. Several complete drafts were generated and reviewed in this manner before a final tentative draft was developed.

This draft was then sent to a panel of experts for outside review. The panel was drawn from officers of the major professional organizations in forensic mental health (i.e., American Academy of Psychiatry and Law; Commission on the Mentally Disabled, American Bar Association; Division of Psychology and Law, American Psychological Association; American Psychology-Law Society). In addition, a panel of Virginia attorneys and judges was asked to review the test to ensure validity in assessing knowledge of relevant Virginia law. The panels of experts unanimously concluded that the test reflected a comprehensive, representative sample of knowledge important in criminal justice and forensic evaluation. Only minor editorial revision was necessary before administering the test to the experimental groups.[2]

Impact of Forensic Training on Level of Relevant Knowledge

To evaluate the impact of training on level of forensic knowledge, we compared the performance of the trainees on the examination with that of several control groups.

METHOD

The forensic knowledge examination was administered to the twenty-seven trainees from the experimental (E) clinics six to eight weeks after the completion of training. The trainees were aware that successful performance on the examination would determine whether they received the certificate indicating that they had adequately completed their forensic training. The examinations also were administered to several control groups. Primary among these was a director-designee group (referred to as the designees), consisting of four or five staff members selected by their clinic director from each of the comparison (C) clinics. As described in chapter 2, the clinic directors were asked to designate those individuals who *would have* composed the prospective forensic team and taken the training, had their clinic been among the E clinics.

We hypothesized that selecting the direct control group in this way would maximize the comparability between groups. To test this hypothesis, we compared the trainees and designees with respect to their professional degrees, disciplines, clinic responsibilities, and previous forensic training. All valid comparisons were nonsignificant. The groups did not differ with respect to the relative frequency of master's versus doctoral professionals, χ^2 (1, $N = 54$) = 2.30, $p = .13$; professionals with training in medicine, psychology, and social work, χ^2 (2, $N = 55$) = 2.36, $p = .31$; or professionals involved primarily in the provision of direct clinical service versus administration, training, or other functions,

2. After careful consideration, we decided not to include a copy of the test itself in this volume. A revised version of the test continues to be used as one important criterion of trainees' successful completion of the forensic training program. The Institute of Law, Psychiatry and Public Policy continues to train community mental health professionals in the state and will continue to do so for some time in the future. Therefore, the publication of the test would violate test security and make it impossible for this test to be used as a criterion in the future. This decision on our part makes it impossible for us to publish item-related analyses, which we performed.

Copies of the examination will be made available, however, to investigators wishing to use it in research or to coordinators of related programs who wish to use it as an evaluative measure.

$\chi^2 (1, N = 54) = .02, p = .88$. A valid chi-square test could not be performed on the values indicating previous level of forensic training because of the high number of cells with zero or low values. However, a visual examination of the data reveals that of the fifty-five individuals, two designees and no trainees had *previous* forensic training of any type.

Examinations also were administered to the remainder of the staff in both the $E (N = 42)$ and $C (N = 46)$ mental health centers. Comparing the performances of the trainees with the other groups was expected to identify further the effects of the forensic training on the level of knowledge of the trainees, because we would not otherwise predict differences in level of forensic knowledge between the trainees and their colleagues, particularly the designees. Comparisons of the degrees, disciplines, and professional roles of trainees, designees, and other staff from the E and C clinics revealed that the latter group included a higher proportion of master's-level mental health professionals, $\chi^2 (3, N = 144) = 11.63, p < .01$. This finding would suggest that trainees and designees may be comparable regarding level and type of professional training and have a higher level of training than other clinic staff.

Even if the trainees were to perform at a level superior to that of the designees and other community mental health professionals on the forensic knowledge examination, it would not reveal whether the trainees' level of knowledge was sufficiently sophisticated to meet with more generalizable criteria delineating expertise in forensic psychology. Thus, we also compared the trainees with a nationally recognized criterion group, the American Board of Forensic Psychology (ABFP). The examination was sent to fifty-four diplomates of the board[3] (i.e., the entire board, excluding persons who had served as reviewers or consultants in the development of the examination). The purpose of the research was explained to the diplomates, who were asked to complete the exam and return it anonymously. Thirty-one diplomates responded, although only twenty-seven were included in the data analyses. The remaining four were trained in specialties of forensic psychology other than criminal and juvenile law (e.g., health policy) and therefore would not have been comparable to the trainees. The questions pertaining to Virginia law were deleted from the examination given to the ABFP since there was no expectation that these professionals would have access to that knowledge base.

The examination also was administered to fifty-three trial judges from a broad range of jurisdictions across the United States. These judges were attending seminars sponsored by the American Academy of Judicial Education

3. Diplomates of the American Board of Forensic Psychology must be licensed, doctoral-level psychologists with a minimum of five years' experience in forensic psychology. They must pass an oral examination administered by a three-member committee prior to admission to diplomate status.

held at the University of Virginia School of Law during the summer of 1981. The judges were administered the modified version of the examination, with the Virginia legal questions deleted. There was no assumption on our part about this group's representativeness of any national or local population. However, we hoped that the performance of the judges on the examination would provide us the opportunity for some initial exploration of the baseline levels of forensic mental health knowledge which such a sample of judges demonstrates. (Further information about the background of these judges is presented in chapter 5.)

RESULTS

Two multivariate analyses of variance (MANOVAs) were performed to compare the examination scores of four groups from community mental health centers: the trainees, the director-designees, the nontrainees from the E clinics (referred to as nontrainees^E), and the non–director-designees from the C clinics (referred to as nondesignees^C). As noted above, the eighty-item examination had been developed to cover the following substantive areas: general forensic issues, competency to stand trial, mental state at the time of the offense, sentencing, and juvenile law. For each module, there was coverage of relevant national law, Virginia law, clinical issues, and research issues. The two MANOVAs permitted examination of the test scores according to these two breakdowns or subgroupings of the same items. We recognize the nonindependence of these two tests. However, we felt that the qualitative information obtained by performing both sets of analyses was valuable to this investigation because, if the results of the MANOVAs were statistically significant, they would allow the performance of univariate tests revealing the content areas in which the groups differed.

The results of both MANOVAs were highly significant. Where the dependent variables were general forensic, competency, mental state at the time of the offense, sentencing, and juvenile issues (subgrouping I), the level of significance was $p < .001$, $F (15, 376) = 10.00$. Where the dependent variables were national legal, Virginia legal, clinical issues, and research issues (subgrouping II), the level of significance also was less than .001, $F (12, 363) = 11.86$. We therefore performed univariate tests to determine which of the content item groupings accounted for these differences. All tests revealed differences among groups significant at the .0001 level, general forensic, $F (3, 140) = 24.23$; competency, $F (3, 140) = 39.02$; mental state, $F (3, 140) = 31.01$; sentencing, $F (3, 140) = 13.04$; juvenile, $F (3, 140) = 28.59$; national legal, $F (3, 140) = 25.48$; Virginia legal, $F (3, 140) = 43.04$; clinical issues, $F (3, 140) = 36.60$; research issues, $F (3, 140) = 17.37$. Means and standard deviations are

Table 4: Forensic Examination Subtest and Total Scores:
Means, Standard Deviations, and Total Mean Percentages Correct

	Trainees N = 27		Director-Designees N = 28		Nontrainees from Experimental Clinics N = 43		Non-Director-Designees from Control Clinics N = 46	
	M	SD	M	SD	M	SD	M	SD
Subgrouping I (Max. Score = 20)								
National Legal	16.63	2.56	11.71	2.80	12.54	2.38	11.67	2.48
Virginia Legal	13.63	3.13	7.25	2.47	7.72	1.83	7.15	2.90
Clinical Issues	17.07	1.66	12.29	2.72	12.51	2.25	11.33	2.50
Research Issues	12.41	3.00	8.21	2.41	9.00	2.56	8.00	2.72
Subgrouping II (Max. Score = 16)								
General Forensic	11.82	2.39	8.00	2.16	8.05	2.32	7.59	1.96
Competency	13.52	1.95	7.79	1.91	9.30	2.34	8.39	2.42
MSO	11.70	2.58	7.11	2.17	7.61	1.62	7.11	2.32
Sentencing	10.70	2.07	8.18	1.96	8.77	1.65	7.85	2.14
Juvenile Law	12.00	2.09	8.39	1.75	8.05	2.01	7.22	2.62
Examination Total Scores								
Total Raw Score (Maximum = 80)	59.74	8.76	39.46	6.84	41.77	5.98	38.15	7.86
Mean Percentage Correct (Maximum = 100%)	74.68		49.33		52.21		47.69	

Table 5: Forensic Examination Subtest and Total Scores: Means, Standard Deviations, and Total Mean Percentages Correct

	Trainees N = 27		Director-Designees N = 28		Judges N = 52		American Board of Forensic Psychology N = 27	
	M	SD	M	SD	M	SD	M	SD
Subgrouping I (Max. Score = 20)								
National Legal	16.63	2.56	11.71	2.80	14.13	2.98	15.85	2.20
Clinical Issues	17.07	1.66	12.29	2.72	7.71	2.64	14.52	2.44
Research Issues	12.41	3.00	8.21	2.41	8.06	2.41	10.93	3.01
Subgrouping II (Max. Score = 12)								
General Forensic	8.78	1.74	6.43	1.75	6.86	1.17	8.93	1.49
Competency	10.33	1.44	6.25	1.67	6.56	2.10	8.56	2.01
MSO	8.96	1.97	6.21	2.31	6.05	2.17	8.63	2.31
Sentencing	8.89	1.53	7.04	1.79	5.27	1.88	8.37	1.42
Juvenile Law	9.15	1.54	6.29	1.36	5.15	2.02	6.81	1.86
Total Test (Max. Score = 60)	46.11	6.44	32.21	5.84	29.90	6.29	41.30	6.49
Total Percentage Correct	76.85		53.68		49.83		68.83	

Note: The items pertaining specifically to Virginia law (*n* = 20) were not administered to the judges and American Board of Forensic Psychology since there was no expectation that these two groups would have access to such knowledge. Thus, these items were omitted from the analyses reported here.

reported in Table 4. Contrasts revealed that the level of forensic knowledge acquired by the trainees was significantly higher ($p < .001$) than that of the other groups, which did not differ significantly from one another.

Similar tests were performed in comparing the following groups: trainees, designees, diplomates (of the ABFP), and the trial judges. The MANOVAs performed with both subgroupings of scores were statistically significant: subgrouping I, $F (15, 348) = 12.83, p < .001$; subgrouping II, $F (9, 312) = 31.99, p < .001$. These analyses did not include items identified as Virginia legal. Univariate analyses revealed differences on each scale: general forensic, $F (3, 130) = 22.66, p < .0001$; competency, $F (3, 130) = 31.50, p < .0001$; mental state, $F (3, 130) = 16.24, p < .0001$; sentencing, $F (3, 130) = 34.52, p < .0001$; juvenile, $F (3, 130) = 30.38, p < .0001$; national legal, $F (3, 130) = 17.88, p < .0001$; clinical issues, $F (3, 130) = 101.22, p < .0001$; research issues, $F (3, 130) = 20.51, p < .0001$. Means and standard deviations are reported in Table 5.

Contrasts performed with the modified multiple range test revealed that the total examination scores of the trainee and diplomate groups were significantly higher than those of the designee and trial judge groups, $p < .001$. This pattern of group differences was also found for the following item groupings: general forensic, competency, mental state, and research issues. For the sentencing and clinical groupings, the trainees performed significantly better than the designees and the trial judges, and both the diplomates and the designees performed better than the trial judges, $p < .001$. For the juvenile law groupings, the trainees earned significantly higher scores than all other groups, and the diplomates performed significantly better than the trial judges, $p < .001$. In the national legal groupings, the trainees, diplomates, and trial judges achieved significantly higher scores than the designees, $p < .001$. (The alpha level for the contrasts was set at a stringent criterion—.001—to reduce the likelihood of spurious findings, given the large number of tests performed and the noninde-pendence of the two subgroupings.)

DISCUSSION

The results strongly suggest that the forensic training offered to Virginia community mental health professionals by the Institute of Law, Psychiatry and Public Policy allowed the program trainees to acquire a level of forensic knowledge superior to that demonstrated by their nonforensically trained counterparts: the director-designees. The trainees achieved a mean percentage of test items correct of approximately 75 percent, whereas the designees earned a mean score of approximately 50 percent. The nontrainees[E] and the nondesignees[C] also performed at about the 50 percent level. Thus, despite the somewhat higher percentage of master's-level versus doctoral-level personnel in these latter groups, their level of forensic knowledge is fairly similar to that demonstrated by the director-designees. In addition, no "spillover" effect was observed in the *E* clinics. One might have expected that the increased sophistication of the trainees regarding forensic matters might lead to increased levels of knowledge among their nontrainee colleagues, resulting from communication among staff members and the new forensic services offered by the clinics. However, no such effect was measured by the examination scores.

The differences among the four groups of Virginia community mental health professionals were consistent across all categories of item groupings. This finding suggests that the training was successful in imparting a level of expert knowledge in all of the content areas included.

However, it is not sufficient to demonstrate that the trainees are superior to their nonforensically trained peers. Although this relative comparison is crucial for evaluating the effect of the training on level of forensic knowledge, it does not tell us how the level of forensic knowledge exhibited by the trainees compares with that of recognized forensic mental health experts. Therefore, we compared the scores of the trainees with those of the diplomates of the ABFP. As the results in Table 5 indicate, the total examination scores of the trainees and the diplomates did not differ significantly. In addition, the analyses of the component groupings indicate that these two groups differed significantly on only one category—juvenile law—in which the trainees performed somewhat better than the diplomates. This finding is logical, however. Regardless of the trainees' background as clinicians working specifically with adults or children, all participated in training on juvenile forensic issues. By contrast, such exposure does not necessarily characterize the training of the typical forensic expert, who may receive little or no exposure to juvenile forensic issues. Data provided by the diplomates who completed the examination revealed that over 50 percent are either not involved or are rarely involved in juvenile cases. This probably explains their lower scores on the juvenile law items.

The findings strongly support the conclusion that through forensic training the trainees acquired a level of forensic knowledge superior to that of their nonforensically trained peers and commensurate with a nationally recognized criterion group: the ABFP.

General Level of Forensic Knowledge among Mental Health Professionals

An interesting, and unexpected, finding of this research is the apparent equivalence in the levels of forensic knowledge demonstrated by several groups of nonforensically trained mental health professionals. As one can observe from

Table 4, the three comparison groups all achieved a mean percentage of approximately 50. Further, the subtest scores were similar across groups.

Some additional data provide even more support for the notion of a normative level of forensic knowledge among mental health professionals. The clinical faculty of the department of behavioral medicine and psychiatry at the University of Virginia were asked to complete the examination, as were the psychology and psychiatry fellows and residents. We hoped these groups could serve as comparison groups of university-based, nonforensically trained mental health professionals. Unfortunately, the response rate was quite poor—about 25 percent. Thus, the data were not included in the analyses. However, a perusal of the means reveals that university-based mental health professionals achieved scores strikingly similar to those of the other nonforensically trained mental health professionals. The clinical faculty ($N = 8$) earned a mean percentage of 51.88, and the residents and fellows ($N = 9$) earned a mean percentage of 52.92.

These observations clearly suggest that a baseline level of forensic knowledge is acquired by most mental health professionals in the course of their training and early career experience. Because the residents and fellows have had relatively limited clinical experience, we speculate that the core of this knowledge may be acquired through training and early exposure rather than through extensive clinical experience, although continued clinical experience may update this basic knowledge. The acquisition of a basic core of forensic knowledge does not appear specific to community mental health work, since university-based personnel demonstrate a similar level of knowledge (although, admittedly, the university sample from which we are generalizing is small). Further, examination performance did not appear to vary with the prevalence of master's- versus doctoral-level professionals. The nontrainee[E] and nondesignee[C] groups had larger proportions of master's-level mental health professionals than did the director-designee or university-based groups, yet the exam scores remained similar. To test this further, we compared the total examination scores of examinees with master's-level versus doctoral-level degrees in psychology with a MANOVA. Included in this sample were the various community mental health center and University of Virginia groups. No significant differences were found, $F (4, 53) = 1.19$, $p = .33$.

Forensic Knowledge among Trial Judges

Comparisons of the examination scores of the trainees, designees, diplomates, and trial judges were perhaps the most interesting. As noted above, the trainees and diplomates demonstrated higher overall levels of forensic knowledge than the designees and trial judges. The judges, like the mental health professionals, achieved a mean percentage score of approximately 50. However, the pattern of group differences in the *subtest* scores was of particular interest. The trainees and diplomates were superior in forensic knowledge to the trial judges except in one grouping: national legal. This finding is perhaps intuitively obvious. One would expect, or hope, that trial judges would demonstrate a level of expertise about the law relating to forensic mental health issues that is higher than that of forensic mental health experts and nonforensically trained mental health professionals. This pattern of differences was observed for the national legal items. One would also expect that nonforensically trained mental health clinicians would evidence a significantly higher level of knowledge about clinical forensic material than judges, who are attorneys, although not as high a level as forensically trained clinicians. Again, this pattern was observed.

With respect to the research issues subgrouping, the trainees and diplomates performed significantly better than the judges and designees, who obtained similar scores on research issues. This finding is logical in that one would not necessarily expect nonforensically trained community mental health clinicians to evidence a higher level of forensic knowledge relating to social science issues than trial judges. The nonforensically trained clinicians, only a proportion of whom are doctoral-level psychologists, may have had little research training. As contrasted with clinical knowledge, one would not expect that these individuals would acquire such scientific knowledge in the course of their training and careers.

The patterns of differences among subtest scores were less revealing when the examination was grouped according to the substantive content areas (i.e., subgrouping I) because the judges performed more poorly than the trainees and diplomates in all cases and more poorly than the designees in one case. Only when the items were grouped according to disciplinary areas of specialization (i.e., law, clinical work, research) were differential patterns of scores observed.

Conclusions

The performance of the sample groups on the specialized examination of forensic knowledge leads to several conclusions. First, concentrated and intensive training in forensic mental health can raise the level of forensic knowledge of community mental health professionals above that of their nonforensically trained colleagues. Second, the level of forensic knowledge acquired by the trainees is comparable to the level demonstrated by a national criterion group of forensic experts, which suggests that the trainees have attained a sufficient level of expertise by national standards. Third, mental health professionals working within the community and academic settings may typically acquire a basic level of knowledge about forensic mental health issues without formal training. That level appears to be relatively consistent across work settings and degree levels. Fourth, overall, the level of forensic knowledge of the trainees and national forensic experts is superior to that of a sample of trial judges. Forensic mental health experts may have a level of expertise, or specialized knowledge, that trial judges do not—that is, they are significantly more knowledgeable about clinical information and behavioral science data in forensic mental health. However, the trial judges in our sample did not differ significantly from the forensic mental health experts within the one specialty area where they would be expected to maintain an adequate level of knowledge: national legal forensic issues.

These findings provide further support for the practicality and effectiveness of the community-based system of forensic services. In addition to reducing forensic evaluation admissions and concomitant costs, the pilot program appears to have been successful in training forensic clinicians who later were capable of demonstrating an adequate level of forensic knowledge. These comparisons provide evidence for the quality of the services provided by the forensic trainees. Level of knowledge is a fundamental dimension of competence; however, some measure of the trainees' actual performance as forensic clinicians also must be conducted before one concludes that the program has been successful. Chapter 4 reviews the findings of the report quality study, which was an attempt to provide such a behavioral measure.

The Quality of Community-Based Forensic Services

The community mental health professionals who had participated in a training program offered at the University of Virginia demonstrated a level of relevant forensic knowledge superior to that of their nonforensically trained colleagues, superior to that of a sample of judges, and equivalent to that of a sample of national experts in forensic psychology. We expect the acquisition of relevant forensic knowledge to be a prerequisite to providing competent forensic evaluation services. In this chapter, we examine the level of skill demonstrated by the trained community mental health professionals as they apply their knowledge to the preparation of forensic evaluation reports. We also review the findings regarding the quality of community-based services from a brief survey of legal professionals who are using them.

The reports submitted to the courts and legal professionals by forensic mental health clinicians are tangible products of this evaluation. The report and subsequent elaboration through testimony in some instances serve to communicate the professional's observations, impressions, and findings to legal professionals and juries. As such, the report must not only reflect a high-quality clinical assessment but also convey the findings in a manner that is clear, comprehensible, free from bias and distortion, focused on the relevant legal questions and criteria, and that presents to the reader the factual and clinical material that led to their conclusions.

Unfortunately, as Roesch and Golding (1980) point out, most forensic evaluation reports do not meet these criteria. "Current reports are most frequently stereotyped in form, often containing only summary conclusions (defendant is competent) or relatively abstract psychiatric phraseology (defendant showed evidence of persecutory delusions). The psychiatric community has a well-deserved reputation for testifying in conclusory, mystique-producing ways, clouding the real uncertainties of their conclusions" (p. 83). Roesch and Golding continue by citing Bazelon (1975): "Psychiatrists have never been able to understand that conclusory labels and opinions are no substitute for facts derived from disciplined investigation" (p. 181).

The forensic mental health training offered by the Institute of Law, Psychiatry and Public Policy schooled participants in the preparation of forensic evaluation reports which, it was hoped, would provide legal professionals with meaningful and comprehensible data. These reports did *not* emphasize the conclusory opinions that so frequently typify the courtroom contributions of clinicians. The model forensic evaluation report used in the training is described below.

Model Forensic Evaluation Reports

Principle 1f of the *Ethical Principles of Psychologists* (American Psychological Association, 1981) states: "As practitioners, psychologists know that they bear a heavy social responsibility because their recommendations and professional actions may alter the lives of others." This reality is perhaps best exemplified in forensic psychology, where the findings of a psychologist can have an impact on events as far reaching as whether a defendant will be imprisoned and, if so, for how long, or whether a defendant will receive the death penalty. In non-criminal spheres of forensic work, psychologists' evaluations may influence whether an allegedly abused or neglected child is removed from the home, whether a child lives with a mother or father after divorce, or whether a mentally disabled person is sterilized. Psychologists who provide such clinical courtroom consultation must perform their evaluation with an exemplary level of competence, responsibility, and awareness of the ramifications of their behavior.

Given the serious consequences that follow the submission of any forensic evaluation, we believe that several rules must be followed by clinicians in the preparation of forensic evaluation reports.

SEPARATION OF FACT FROM OPINION

In the course of a forensic evaluation, the examiner will collect data from several sources: interviews with involved parties, written records, observation of the subject(s) of the evaluation, possibly the administration of psychological tests, and so forth. The information gathered during the course of the evaluation will be interpreted and organized by the clinician in a manner consistent with his or her training, theoretical orientation, and perspectives. What emerges at the end of this process is not the *truth* about the issues in question but an *opinion* by one clinician or a team of clinicians about the issues in question. The weight given to the opinion by the trier of fact will be a product of many variables, which perhaps may be related to the perceived competence of the clinician or the persuasiveness of the clinician's analysis of the data. However, the reality remains: the findings of each clinician are merely opinions, which may be similar to or different from the conclusions drawn by any other clinician interpreting the same raw data. Each clinician, then, must separate for the trier of fact and relevant parties in a case what is fact and what is inference, interpretation, or opinion.

Facts, such as statements made by individuals, or information derived from written records must be attributed to their source. Thus, the report should not include unattributed statements such as this: "Mr. Smith performed poorly in school." Rather, such information should be attributed to the source providing it: "Mr. Smith reported that he had performed poorly in school," or "The court's social history report indicates that Mr. Smith failed and was retained several grades in school." Sections of an evaluation report providing background information and descriptions of the defendant's behavior during the interview should include no unattributed statements and no inferences of any type. Subsequent sections of the report, labeled appropriately as 'Clinical Impressions," "Clinical Formulation," "Clinical Findings," or "Opinion," should be the repository of all such inferential and interpretive material. The separation of factual and inferential material in a forensic evaluation report may be seen as analogous to the separation in scientific papers in psychology of results and subsequent discussion (i.e., interpretation) of those results.

PRESENTATION OF THE FACTUAL BASIS OF ONE'S OPINIONS
For the reasons specified above, it is not only crucial to separate and label facts and inference or opinion, but it is also essential that the clinician present to the reader how he or she applied and interpreted the factual material in reaching the opinion. In so doing, the clinician provides the trier of fact, or the legal professionals representing the parties in the case, with the opportunity to accept or reject the clinician's analysis of the data.

Most important, the determination of the ultimate legal issue will be made by the trier of fact, not by the clinician. That is, to the degree that the trier of fact has access to the raw data and has an understanding of the clinician's process of interpretation of that data, the trier of fact is better situated to make an educated decision regarding how much reliance to place on the evaluation report. To the extent that the trier of fact is forced to accept or reject an expert's opinion without having insight into the basis of those judgments, the influence of the expert may be lessened or inappropriately increased.

FOCUS ON RELEVANT AND APPROPRIATE LEGAL ISSUES
A forensic evaluation report differs from a diagnostic report or intellectual evaluation because the questions addressed in the forensic evaluation are defined by the legal system, not by the mental health or educational system. In making this transition, some clinical consultants to the courts are unable to adjust ap-

propriately the focus and format of their evaluations and reports. For example, in the case of competency to stand trial, legal criteria require that a defendant be capable of understanding the proceedings against him and of participating in his defense.[1] Whereas information about diagnosis and intellectual level may be relevant to capacity along those dimensions, such information does not directly address the legal questions. Examination of the questions of interest to the law require an evaluation strategy that is criterion-relevant and focused on the specific aspects of behavior and functioning, which are in question.

A good forensic evaluation report reveals that the clinician knew and applied the relevant legal standards in the course of the evaluation and that the evaluation procedures were appropriate to the questions raised by the specific type of evaluation. In addition, a good forensic evaluation report provides a minimum of superfluous information. This is important for brevity and for preserving the defendant's right to have little or no extraneous information about his background and functioning revealed in a forensic evaluation report.

CLARITY OF WRITING

Finally, to make the report as comprehensible as possible, clinicians are encouraged to define any terms of art or diagnostic terms (e.g., "characterological," "psychotic") and to write in an unambiguous and clear manner to non–mental health professionals. Again, writing in such a manner may be new to most clinicians. However, to assure that the findings of an evaluator will be considered fully and interpreted properly, they must be comprehensible. Some clinicians may strive to impress and perhaps confuse a jury with their use of multisyllabic psychological jargon, but this approach serves to impede rather than facilitate the search for truth that is the aim of legal proceedings. An appropriate compromise for the expert is to demonstrate his or her knowledge of the field through occasional use of the jargon but in all instances to define those terms so as to ensure that the meaning of the report is comprehended fully.

The outline format used in the forensic evaluation training of the Institute of Law, Psychiatry and Public Policy for reports on competency to stand trial is presented in appendix C.

The Report Quality Study

METHOD

We examined the quality of the forensic evaluations performed by the community clinicians. In Virginia, the courts had long relied on forensic evaluation re-

1. Dusky v. United States, 362 U.S. 402 (1960).

ports prepared by the experts staffing the forensic unit of one of the major state hospitals. This forensic unit was the primary site of forensic evaluations in Virginia until the onset of the community-based and hospital outpatient program. Thus, we deemed the reports prepared by the personnel of this unit to be an appropriate criterion against which to evaluate the reports prepared by the community program's trainees.

At the end of the pilot year of the community-based program, we obtained forensic evaluation reports from the six experimental clinics and from the forensic unit at the state hospital. The community mental health center reports had been prepared during the pilot year of the program (March 1, 1981, to February 28, 1982), but the reports obtained from the forensic unit had been prepared prior to July 1, 1981, because early in July 1981, the staff of the forensic unit, as part of the development of the new hospital-based outpatient program, participated in the forensic training offered by the Institute of Law, Psychiatry and Public Policy. Subsequent to that training, their report format was altered to reflect the model suggested in the training. Thus, so as not to contaminate the comparison between the community trainees and forensic unit experts, only pre–July 1981 hospital reports were included in the study.

Reports were randomly selected from each of the facilities within three categories of report: competency to stand trial, mental state at the time of the offense, and presentence. The reports were then "sanitized" so that all information identifying individuals, locales, evaluation facilities, specific courts, and so forth was replaced with fictitious identifiers. In addition, phraseology that would reveal whether the evaluation had been performed on an inpatient or outpatient basis (e.g., "Mr. Smith came into the clinic for two appointments") was deleted. The reports were retyped by our staff on plain paper. All of these steps were taken so that raters could be blind to the source of the report and to protect the confidentiality of the client.

The panel of expert raters consisted of three judges, three prosecuting attorneys, and three defense attorneys. The individuals were selected to serve on this panel because of their esteemed reputations within Virginia and for their previous willingness to participate in policy-related efforts in forensic and related matters. Three were from the project's advisory committee (see chapter 6). Most were referred to us by members of the committee. Only one individual (a prosecutor) declined to participate. Because of the extensive amount of time required for reading and rating the reports, these individuals were each offered a modest honorarium (which was refused by one judge who felt that it was part of his public service responsibility to participate in such a project).

Each panel member was sent twenty forensic evaluation reports. Of these reports, eight were competency to stand trial reports (one from each of the six experimental clinics and two from the forensic unit); six were mental state at the time of the offense reports (one from each of four experimental clinics and two from the forensic unit); and six were presentence reports (one from each of four experimental clinics and two from the forensic unit). Two of the experimental clinics had not been engaged in sufficient numbers of mental state at the time of the offense or presentence evaluations to justify inclusion of samples from those categories in the study. Including more reports from the forensic unit would have facilitated further statistical analyses of this data, but because of concern regarding the extensive task being required of raters, we limited the number of reports included in the sample. Representativeness, however, was not viewed as a problem, because the reports generated by the forensic unit were extremely similar to one another, with very little deviation from a standard format.

The raters were sent the twenty reports and three types of rating forms. Each form corresponded to a different type of report: competency to stand trial, mental state at the time of the offense, and presentence. The rating forms were adapted from scales developed by Petrella and Poythress (1983) in their study of interdisciplinary differences in forensic mental health reports. The forms, presented in appendixes D-1, D-2, and D-3, request raters to address issues relating to the quality of each report including use of understandable language, reference to appropriate legal criteria given the type of evaluation, and adequacy of explanation on the basis of the conclusions. Raters were provided with a nine-point scale for each item. They were asked to evaluate each report independently.

RESULTS

Because only two reports of each type prepared by the forensic unit were included in the sample, the number was too small to allow for statistical comparisons between groups for each type of report. However, the final item on the rating scale for each type of report was identical (item G on the report rating forms for competency and mental state at the time of the offense and item H on the presentence report rating form). That item requested a rating of the *overall* quality of the report. Means and standard deviations can be found in Table 6. The ratings of the reports of the forensic unit and clinic reports were compared with separate *t* tests for each category of raters (i.e., judges, defense attorneys, and prosecuting attorneys). The results indicate that all three groups of raters found the clinic reports to be of superior overall quality, with the greatest mean difference observed in the judges' ratings, $t(18) = 4.77, p < .001$, and the defense attorneys' ratings, $t(18) = 4.75, p < .001$. The smallest mean differences were apparent in the ratings of the prosecuting attorneys, $t(18) = 2.91, p < .01$.

62

Table 6: Means and Standard Deviations of Report Quality Ratings on "Overall Quality" Item across All Report Types (Clinics and Central State Hospital)

Rater Group	Clinics (n = 14)		Forensic Unit (n = 6)	
	M	SD	M	SD
Judges**	6.93	1.57	3.39	1.39
Defense Attorneys**	6.71	1.62	3.17	1.28
Prosecuting Attorneys*	6.57	1.32	4.39	1.99

Note: The "Overall Quality" item was item G on the competency and MSO evaluation rating forms, and item H on the presentence evaluation rating forms (1 = poor, 9 = excellent). The three reports were competency evaluation, mental state at the time of the offense evaluation, and presentence evaluation.

*p < .01 **p < .001

The mean responses of the raters on the individual items are reported in Tables 7, 8, and 9, for each type of report, with the rater groups combined. For the competency reports, the mean item ratings for the clinic reports ranged from 6.29 to 7.51, where 5.0 is the midpoint between poor (1.0) and excellent (9.0), and the mean item ratings for the forensic unit reports ranged between 3.06 and 8.06. For reports on the mental state at the time of the offense, the mean item ratings for clinic reports ranged from 7.03 to 7.81, and between 4.28 and 6.44 for the forensic unit reports. Finally, the range was between 6.26 and 7.96 for the clinics and between 1.33 and 7.14 for the forensic unit on the presentence reports.

Table 7: Means and Standard Deviations of Item-by-Item Ratings of Report Quality for Competency Evaluation Reports from Clinics and Central State Hospital (Rater Groups Combined)

Item:	Clinics (n = 6)		Forensic Unit (n = 2)	
	M	SD	M	SD
A	7.51	1.21	8.06	.83
B	7.09	1.26	5.28	1.27
C	6.93	1.76	5.17	2.10
D	6.56	2.01	4.67	1.27
E	6.29	1.76	3.06	1.39
F	6.54	1.76	4.11	1.97
G	6.46	1.62	4.17	1.74

Table 8: Means and Standard Deviations of Item-by-Item Ratings
of Report Quality for Mental State at the Time of the Offense Evaluation Reports
from Clinics and Central State Hospital (Rater Groups Combined)

Item:	Clinics (n = 4)		Forensic Unit (n = 2)	
	M	SD	M	SD
A	7.81	.77	6.44	1.30
B	7.39	1.12	6.25	1.78
C	7.75	.65	4.83	.96
D	7.03	.99	5.64	1.35
E	7.18	.91	4.28	1.42
F	7.25	1.04	4.50	1.30
G	7.26	.98	4.67	1.34

DISCUSSION

The comparison between the clinic and forensic unit reports reveals that all three groups of expert raters considered the reports submitted by the clinics to be superior in overall quality to the forensic unit reports. This evaluation was stronger among the judges and defense attorneys and weaker among the prosecuting attorneys. In all instances, on both the ratings of overall quality and the remaining item ratings, the means of the clinic ratings never fell below 6.26, on a scale where the midpoint was 5.0, and the highest rating is 9.0. The clinic

Table 9: Means and Standard Deviations of Item-by-Item Ratings
of Report Quality for Presentence Evaluation Reports from Clinics
and Central State Hospital (Rater Groups Combined)

Item:	Clinics (n = 4)		Forensic Unit (n = 2)	
	M	SD	M	SD
A	7.96	.78	7.14	1.80
B	7.01	1.71	3.58	1.35
C	7.82	.63	4.75	1.90
D	6.26	1.70	1.50	.59
E	6.58	1.77	1.33	.42
F	6.76	1.91	3.70	2.52
G	6.96	1.74	2.86	1.77
H	6.83	1.53	2.72	1.47

reports were typically viewed as being above average on an absolute scale, while the mean item ratings of the forensic unit reports suggested below average overall quality, with a mix of high and low ratings on the various items.

A further examination of the particular item ratings may shed some light on apparent differences in the ratings by the three groups of legal professionals. A primary difference between the reports prepared by the clinics and the forensic unit is that the former strive to provide the reader with the raw data that led the clinician to his or her conclusions. The latter may do so only incidentally, if at all. Item E on each of the three rating scales addresses this aspect of report writing. On this item the two forensic unit reports were rated most poorly, especially by judges and defense attorneys. Judges, impartial in the search for truth, should seek all and any information that will allow them or the jury to make a knowledgeable judgment in the case. They should favor reports that provide sufficient background and factual information to allow the trier of fact to consider not only the clinician's conclusions but the data that led to those conclusions. Prosecuting attorneys, whose primary aim in a trial may be to convict and obtain a severe sentence for a defendant, may be less positively disposed to a report that provides detailed information about the psychological functioning of a defendant. Such information may make the jury more sympathetic to the defendant, perhaps increasing the likelihood of an insanity acquittal or a milder sentence. Finally, defense attorneys want to differentiate their client from the so-called average offender. The provision of detailed information may serve this end, in their view.

An alternate hypothesis regarding the differences in ratings among legal professionals relates to the degree to which the clinic and hospital reports might be viewed as oriented toward the prosecution or the defense, although this would not explain the higher ratings of the clinic reports by the judges. One might predict that the clinic reports are more sympathetic toward defendants. A perusal of the reports does not support this hypothesis, however. Of the eight reports on competency to stand trial, five of the six clinic reports and the two hospital reports concluded that the defendant appeared to be competent. The sixth clinic report, which focused on a mentally retarded individual, concluded that he was not competent. Of the four reports from clinics on mental state at the time of the offense, only one suggested that the defendant's mental condition had been sufficiently disturbed to warrant consideration by the court in adjudication. (The report indicated that the ultimate decision as to whether the particular disorder and its impact on the alleged criminal behavior met the legal criteria of the insanity defense in Virginia should appropriately be left to the court, and thus it did not state conclusions to that effect.) Of the two reports prepared by the hospital on mental state at the time of the offense, one suggested that the defendant did meet the criteria for the insanity defense in Virginia. Finally, the presentence reports from the hospital staff were rather neutral in tone, as was one of the clinic presentence reports. Two of the clinic presentence reports were extremely unsympathetic toward the defendant, suggesting that the defendant's criminal behavior was ego-syntonic, patterned, and not likely to be ameliorated. The final clinic report was a bit more sympathetic to the defendant, ascribing the criminal behavior to a psychological disorder and problematic life experiences but was pessimistic about rehabilitative potential.

In general, we would conclude that the tone and findings of these reports do not suggest that the clinics were more defense-oriented than the hospitals. This analysis supports our earlier notion that the preference for the clinic reports by the judges and defense attorneys may relate to the depth of information provided in the clinic reports, which allows the court and legal personnel the opportunity to draw their own conclusions from the psychological data and provides them with greater insight into the unique features of the defendant's behavior.

Only on item A were the forensic unit reports typically rated above average. This item relates to the degree to which the reports were understandable. Presentence reports from the forensic unit were rated more poorly than its other reports on most other items.

In general, therefore, it appears that the clinic reports demonstrate relatively consistent high quality and were rated above average in all item categories for each of the three types of reports. In addition, they are rated as superior in quality to the reports prepared by the state hospital's forensic unit, which has, for years, been regarded as the standard within Virginia, because it had served most of the state prior to the onset of the community-based program. It should be noted that the forensic unit reports used in this study are written in the conclusory format that Roesch and Golding (1980) identified as characterizing much mental health testimony. Thus, we propose that the comparisons performed in this study are generalizable to a more basic contrast between the traditional "ultimate issue" conclusory and diagnostic report and the more functionally oriented descriptive report called for by Roesch and Golding (1980) and described earlier in this chapter. As noted above, the forensic experts on the unit participated in the forensic training in July 1981, and since that time reported that they had adopted many of the procedures and report-writing formats recommended by the Institute of Law, Psychiatry and Public Policy. In addition, they are now providing outpatient forensic evaluation services as well and have therefore become proficient in the administration of a brief outpatient forensic interview.

The findings suggest that the level of forensic knowledge apparently acquired by the community-based trainees, as reported in chapter 3, is accompanied by a capacity to apply that knowledge to one's clinical forensic evaluation work. The results reported for these two studies strongly support the notion that community-based services are not only efficient and cost-effective but also provide a higher level of quality in forensic services.

Survey of Legal Professionals within the Experimental Jurisdictions

To supplement the findings reported in this chapter and in chapter 3 regarding the quality of services provided by the experimental clinics, we conducted a brief survey of legal professionals who are actually using the services of community mental health centers.

All district court, circuit court and juvenile court judges within those jurisdictions, all prosecuting attorneys, and three defense attorneys from each jurisdiction were sent a brief survey form in June 1982, approximately fifteen months after the pilot program was initiated. The total sampled was eighty. The professionals were requested to assess the following: the quality of the reports prepared by the community mental health centers, their relationship with the pilot-clinic evaluators in their jurisdictions, and their perception of the general effectiveness of the outpatient evaluation system in meeting the state's forensic evaluation needs. They were asked to rate each item on a five-point scale, where a score of 1.0 represented poor and a score of 5.0 represented excellent.

RESULTS
Forty-nine legal professionals (or 61.25%) responded. Of these respondents, seven indicated that they had not had occasion to use the new forensic evaluation services. The results of this survey appear in Table 10. In most jurisdictions, legal professionals consistently agreed that the quality of services provided by the clinics is high. The one exception to this pattern was jurisdiction A, where two of the seven respondents rated the clinic poor, while five of the respondents rated the clinic high. These two respondents are the district court judges mentioned in chapter 2, who were resistant to the program from its inception.

DISCUSSION
The mean ratings suggest that the legal professionals in the experimental jurisdictions are satisfied with the community-based program. Mean ratings for the six jurisdictions together are all at the level of 4.0 or greater, indicating that the legal professionals consider the services to be of high quality, the community

Table 10: Mean Survey Ratings of Pilot Project by Judges,
Commonwealth's Attorneys, and Defense Attorneys
in Experimental Jurisdictions (Total Respondents = 42)

Jurisdiction	Quality of Reports M	Relationship with Pilot Clinic Evaluators M	General Effectiveness of Outpatient Evaluation System M
A (Number of respondents = 7)	3.57	4.00	3.71
B (Number of respondents = 4)	4.38	4.63	4.38
C (Number of respondents = 3)	4.33	4.00	4.33
D (Number of respondents = 16)	3.50	3.87	3.80
E (Number of respondents = 4)	4.50	4.75	4.50
F (Number of respondents = 8)	3.75	4.50	3.86
Mean Rating	4.01	4.29	4.10

Note: Ratings were on a scale of 1 to 5 where a score of 1 represented "poor" and a score of 5 represented "excellent." A score of 3 therefore was the midpoint, indicating "average" or "satisfactory."

Not included in this table are responses of individuals who did not use the evaluation services ($n = 7$).

mental health professionals to be accessible and easy to work with, and the system to be functioning well in meeting the state's forensic evaluation needs.

This brief survey should not be viewed as a substitute for a more comprehensive evaluation of the perceptions of participants in the program or of the interagency collaborative relationships. A more sophisticated and extensive study of these dimensions of the program is underway. The brief survey was merely an attempt to obtain validation of the findings reported in this chapter and in chapters 2 and 3, by examining the perceptions of the users of the community services.

Given the findings reported in this and the previous two chapters, we find strong support for the notion that efficient, cost-effective community forensic services can be provided without sacrificing quality. Rather, the availability of such community-based services, as we predicted, does appear to allow for the provision of superior services.

Chapter 5

Interaction between Courts and Mental Health Centers

Regardless of the outcome of a program evaluation, it is useful to explore the *processes* that characterize the program. Such an evaluation is useful both for examining the "bugs" in implementing a program (a point which we will discuss in chapter 6) and for developing hypotheses about what may have contributed to the success or failure of a program. This chapter broadly addresses the second point. While examining the processes of the pilot project, we were also able to obtain some interesting data about typical interaction between courts and mental health centers.

Much of the data presented in this chapter is of the most basic time-and-motion variety. We felt that it was important to determine how frequently courts and mental health professionals interact, around what issues, and in what form. Such basic descriptive data about interaction between the mental health and legal systems have heretofore been lacking. We present some initial data, although far from exhaustive, about the quantity and quality of judges' interaction with the mental health professions and of community mental health professionals' involvement in the legal system.

Judges View the Mental Health Professions:
Their Experiences and Attitudes

METHOD

Fifty-three judges attending a judicial education workshop at the University of Virginia in summer 1981 were asked to fill out a questionnaire about their court and their experiences with the mental health system. The participating judges were the same as those in chapter 3 who reported their knowledge of forensic mental health. In addition to providing information about their community and the resources available in their court, the judges responded to a series of questions about the extent of their training, formal and informal, in the behavioral sciences (e.g., psychology, psychiatry, criminology), the frequency with which mental health expertise is introduced on various issues in their court, and their perceptions of the usefulness of such expertise.

Before discussing the results, it is important to note some characteristics of the sample which may affect interpretation of the results. The sample of judges attending the workshop was national; the judges represented twenty-four states and territories. However, regions east of the Mississippi River, especially the Southeast, were overrepresented in the sample. Otherwise, the sample of judges differed, but not markedly so, from national distributions on some key variables. To determine the representativeness of the current sample, we compared it with the sample of judges responding to the questionnaire that Ryan, Ashman, Sales, and Shane-DuBow (1980) sent to all trial judges in state courts in the United States. The results of these comparisons are shown in Table 11. To summarize, the current sample is relatively overrepresented by courts of general jurisdiction in suburban communities. Large courts (more than twenty-five judges) are underrepresented in the sample. The participating judges are also more likely than the national sample to have access to at least one full-time law clerk or a full-time personal secretary.

RESULTS

Training in the Behavioral Sciences. A substantial proportion of the judges (41.5%) reported having attended continuing education workshops on behavioral-science topics. The majority (56.6%) had taken undergraduate courses in the behavioral sciences, but only two (3.8%) had majored in the area. Six (11.3%) had taken related courses in law school. None had obtained a postgraduate degree in the behavioral sciences, and eleven (20.8%) reported no formal training in the behavioral sciences at all.

Many of the judges reported no substantial self-education in behavioral-science topics. The majority (56.6%) reported that they read literature in the field no more than once a year. Only three judges (5.7%) claimed to do such reading at least once a week, and eight others (15.1%) reported reading material in the behavioral sciences at least once a month. Some self-education on major forensic issues is common, however. At least 45 percent reported that they or their clerks had consulted (outside court) a mental health professional, a behavioral scientist, or behavioral-science literature on the following major topic of forensic practice: competency to stand trial, 34 (64.2%); mental state at the time of the offense, 27 (50.9%); amenability to treatment, 25 (47.2%); dangerousness, 30 (56.6%); civil commitment, 23 (43.4%); child custody in divorce, 24 (45.3%); abuse and neglect, 24 (45.3%); other, 7 (13.2%).

Table 11: Characteristics of the Sample of Judges

Work Assignments

Current Study (N = 53)			Ryan et al. (1980) (N = 2,984)		
	n			n	
Appellate	2	(3.8%)	Appellate	3	(0.1%)
Criminal and Civil	34	(64.2%)	General	1,763	(59.1%)
Multiple Assignments	6	(11.2%)			
Juvenile and Domestic			Juvenile	46	(1.5%)
Relations only	2	(3.8%)	Domestic Relations	54	(1.8%)
Criminal only	3	(5.7%)	Criminal only	363	(12.2%)
Civil only	4	(7.5%)	Civil—mixed	631	(21.1%)
			Civil—jury	57	(1.9%)
Other	2	(3.8%)	Probate	18	(0.6%)
			Chancery	41	(1.4%)
			Law and Motions	8	(0.3%)

Region

Current Study[a] (N = 53)		Ryan et al. (1980) (N = 3,032)
9 (17.3%)	Northeast	448 (14.8%)
9 (17.3%)	North Central	998 (32.9%)
30 (57.7%)	South	889 (29.3%)
4 (7.7%)	West	697 (23.0%)

a. No response = 1

Frequency of Mental Health Testimony. A third or more of the judges who hear cases on these issues have testimony or a report by a mental health professional in less than 10 percent of the cases in which such an issue is raised (see Table 12). On the other hand, at least half of the judges reported that such expert opinions were available in more than 90 percent of their cases when the issue is competency to stand trial, mental state at the time of the offense, or civil commitment. Involvement of mental health professionals in domestic relations cases is apparently less common. Clinical testimony or reports are presented in less than 25 percent of the child-custody disputes in the courts of three-fourths

Table 11: *continued*

Community Size[b]

Current Study (N = 53)		Ryan et al. (1980) (N = 2,456)[c]
3 (5.7%)	Large city only (500,000+)	555 (22.6%)
4 (7.5%)	Large city and suburbs (1M+)	
5 (9.4%)	Medium-sized city and suburbs (250,000 to 1M)	366 (14.9%)
14 (26.4%)	Smaller city in nonmetropolitan area (50,000 to 250,000)	652 (26.5%)
10 (18.9%)	Suburban only	175 (7.1%)
17 (32.1%)	Rural	708 (28.8%)

b. $\chi^2(4) = 12.90, p < .02$

Court Size (Number of Judges)[d]

Current Study (N = 53)		Ryan et al. (1980) (N = 2,986)
	Small	
6 (11.3%)	1	436 (14.7%)
12 (22.6%)	2	410 (13.7%)
8 (15.1%)	3–4	430 (14.4%)
	Intermediate	
12 (22.6%)	5–9	485 (16.2%)
8 (15.1%)	10–15	368 (12.3%)
3 (5.7%)	16–25	256 (8.6%)
	Large	
3 (5.7%)	26–39	272 (9.1%)
1 (1.9%)	40 or more	329 (11.0%)

c. Civil judges only

d. $\chi^2(2) = 5.18, p < .10$

(continued)

Table 11: *continued*

Type of Secretarial Services

Current Study (N = 53)		*Ryan et al. (1980)* (N = 2,918)
16 (30.8%)	Court reporter, clerk, or bailiff acts as secretary	951 (32.6%)
4 (7.7%)	Shared, in secretarial pool[e]	431 (14.8%)
2 (3.8%)	Part-time personal secretary	360 (12.3%)
30 (57.7%)	Full-time personal secretary	1,070 (36.7%)
0 (0.0%)	None[f]	106 (3.6%)

Law Clerk Services

Current Study (N = 53)		*Ryan et al. (1980)* (N = 2,993)
2 (3.8%)	> 1 full-time clerk[h]	28 (0.9%)
15 (28.3%)	1 full-time clerk[h]	497 (16.6%)
2 (3.8%)	1 part-time clerk[i]	259 (8.6%)
8 (15.1%)	≥ 1 law-clerk shared[i]	412 (13.8%)
26 (49.1%)	none	1,797 (60.1%)

---

e. Combined for χ^2; $\chi^2(3) = 12.64$, $p < .01$

f. No response by judge in current study = 1

g. $\chi^2(2) = 7.54$, $p < .01$

h. Combined for purposes of computing χ^2

i. Combined for purposes of computing χ^2

of the participating judges; input of mental health professionals is similarly uncommon in the courts of half of the judges when they try cases in which abuse or neglect is alleged. None of the judges have expert opinions of mental health professionals available in more than three-fourths of the custody cases they hear; about one-fourth of the courts have such a high frequency of clinicians' involvement in abuse and neglect cases.

Attitudes toward Mental Health Expertise. On average, judges would apparently like to have the assistance of mental health professionals available more than it is. For each issue, judges identified a report or testimony of a mental health professional as being useful at least more of the time than the expertise was usually available (see Table 13). However, the rank ordering of importance

Table 12: Frequency of Testimony on Reports by Mental Health Professionals

Nature of the Issue		Proportion of Cases					
	Never	<10%	<25%	<50%	<75%	<90%	>90%
Competency to stand trial	1 (2.1%)	15 (31.3%)	3 (6.3%)	2 (4.2%)	1 (2.5%)	2 (4.2%)	24 (50.0%)
Mental state at time of the offense	1 (2.0%)	16 (32.7%)	1 (2.0%)	2 (4.1%)	0 (0.0%)	3 (6.1%)	26 (53.1%)
Amenability to treatment	4 (8.7%)	15 (32.6%)	0 (0.0%)	4 (8.7%)	4 (8.7%)	0 (0.0%)	19 (41.3%)
Dangerousness	2 (4.3%)	18 (39.1%)	1 (2.2%)	6 (13.0%)	1 (2.2%)	1 (2.2%)	17 (37.0%)
Civil commitment	5 (11.1%)	9 (20.0%)	3 (6.7%)	1 (2.2%)	1 (2.2%)	0 (0.0%)	26 (57.8%)
Child custody in divorce	4 (10.0%)	18 (45.0%)	8 (20.0%)	5 (12.5%)	5 (12.5%)	0 (0.0%)	0 (0.0%)
Child abuse and neglect	5 (11.9%)	11 (26.2%)	5 (11.9%)	10 (23.8%)	1 (2.4%)	5 (11.9%)	5 (11.9%)

Note: $N = 53$; n's equal less than 53 because of blanks and "not applicable" responses (i.e., participating judge does not hear cases on this issue).

Table 13: Judicial Attitudes toward the Involvement of Mental Health Professionals

Nature of the Issue	Judges' Perceptions of Usefulness					
	Never Useful	Seldom Useful	Occasionally Useful	Often Useful	Useful Most of the Time	Essential
Competency to stand trial	1 (2.0%)	0 (0.0%)	1 (2.0%)	4 (8.0%)	10 (20.0%)	34 (68.0%)
Mental state at the time of the offense	1 (2.0%)	1 (2.0%)	0 (0.0%)	7 (14.0%)	15 (30.0%)	26 (52.0%)
Amenability to treatment	6 (11.8%)	3 (5.9%)	3 (5.9%)	6 (11.8%)	18 (35.3%)	15 (29.4%)
Dangerousness	5 (10.0%)	2 (4.0%)	1 (2.0%)	4 (8.0%)	22 (44.0%)	16 (32.0%)
Civil commitment	7 (13.5%)	1 (1.9%)	3 (5.8%)	1 (1.9%)	7 (13.5%)	33 (63.5%)
Child custody	8 (16.7%)	3 (6.3%)	11 (22.9%)	8 (16.7%)	14 (29.2%)	4 (8.3%)
Abuse and neglect	6 (12.5%)	5 (10.4%)	6 (12.5%)	6 (12.5%)	16 (33.3%)	9 (18.8%)

Note: $N = 53$; n's equal less than 53 because of blanks.

of mental health testimony roughly paralleled the relative frequency of actual presentation of such testimony. Thus, about half identified mental health professionals' input in domestic relations cases as useful at least most of the time (child custody, 37.5%; abuse and neglect, 52.1%)

Attitudes differed toward mental health professionals in the courtroom (see Table 14). For example, attitudes regarding the usefulness of mental health professionals in issues related to the adjudication of criminal cases (i.e., competency to stand trial, mental state at the time of the offense) loaded on a separate factor, eigenvalue = 2.44. These attitudes are moderately correlated with attitudes toward clinicians' involvement in issues related to sentencing and not correlated at all with attitudes toward clinicians' involvement on civil issues. Similarly, there is a substantial correlation between perceptions of the usefulness of clinicians' opinions about amenability to treatment and similar attitudes about clinical predictions of dangerousness, both issues arising at sentencing.

Relationships among Variables. None of the variables strongly differentiated courts where judges rarely hear opinions of mental health professionals. For example, community size was unrelated to the frequency of mental health input on any of the seven forensic issues noted on the questionnaire. There were highly significant correlations between attitudes toward use of mental health professionals and the reported frequency of clinicians' appearance in their

Table 14: Relationships among Judicial Attitudes
toward the Involvement of Mental Health Professionals

	Nature of the Issue						
	CTST	MSO	ATT	DANG	CIVCOM	CUST	A/N
CTST	—	.81***	.28*	.34**	.19	.12	−.10
MSO	.81***	—	.34**	.15	.21	.20	−.02
ATT	.28*	.34**	—	.62***	.39**	.30*	.25*
DANG	.34**	.15	.62***	—	.27*	.28*	.27*
CIVCOM	.19	.21	.39**	.27*	—	.24*	.24*
CUST	.12	.20	.30*	.28*	.24*	—	.42**
A/N	−.10	−.02	.25*	.27*	.24*	.42**	—

CTST = competency to stand trial, MSO = mental state at the time of the offense, ATT = amenability to treatment, DANG = dangerousness, CIVCOM = civil commitment, CUST = child custody in divorce, A/N = abuse and neglect

*$p < .05$ **$p < .01$ ***$p < .0001$

courts with respect to sentencing and civil issues, $r = .50$ to .56, but not with respect to competency to stand trial, $r = .21$, or mental state at the time of the offense, $r = .08$.

The court-structure and training variables also failed to provide significant explanation of the variance in judges' attitudes toward the mental health professions. Among the various training variables, the only statistically significant result was a weak correlation ($r = .24$) between the frequency with which judges read behavioral-science literature and their perceptions of the importance of mental health experts' opinions in determining defendants' mental state at the time of the offense. Given the number of correlations considered, this single finding may have been by chance and nevertheless accounts for minimal variance.

Court resources may affect the *opportunity* for judges to be influenced by the behavioral sciences, however. The frequency with which judges reported reading behavioral-science material was highly related to the level of secretarial services available, $r = .72, p < .001$, although unrelated to the size of the court (number of judges), $r = -.01$, or the availability of law clerks, $r = .21$. Judges in nonmetropolitan communities were more likely than their metropolitan colleagues to read behavioral-science literature no more than once a year, $\chi^2 (1) = 10.06, p < .01$.

DISCUSSION

Judicial Attitudes. The results of this study suggest that the typical trial judge lacks substantial foundation and perhaps interest in the behavioral sciences. In view of the explicitly psychological goals of many of their functions, especially in criminal law, this finding is somewhat surprising. It does, however, corroborate our conclusion in chapter 3 that mental health professionals are likely to possess specialized knowledge unavailable to the trier of fact.

Judges apparently share the latter view, because they reported a belief in the usefulness of mental health professionals in the legal system. There may be a mismatch between judges' expectations and the expertise of mental health professionals, however. Notably, 76 percent of the participants reported that they believed clinicians' opinions on dangerousness to be useful at least most of the time. In that regard, the low validity of such assessments has been well chronicled (see, e.g., Monahan, 1981). At the same time, though, the judges showed substantially less faith in clinicians' ability to assist in cases of child custody and abuse and neglect. Clearly mental health professionals generally feel much more comfortable in discussing family relations, a matter with which they deal constantly and about which there is a large body of research (see, e.g., Hetherington & Martin, 1979). One wonders whether the misplaced judicial emphasis is simply a matter of "passing the buck" on hard questions or if it is primarily thinking of mental health law as being "medical."[1]

In all fairness, however, judges' relative lack of confidence in clinicians' potential contributions to family law cases may be well founded. Virtually no research directly assesses the effects of various custody dispositions (Clingempeel & Reppucci, 1982; Melton, 1984). Moreover, mental health professionals assessing children's "best interests" may focus on questions of "psychological parenthood" (cf. Goldstein, Freud, & Solnit, 1973) to the exclusion of issues of parental "responsibility" which may enter into the legal calculus (Lowery, 1981).

Contacts with the Mental Health System. Regardless of the level of sophistication that judges bring to contacts with mental health professionals, one of the most curious findings of the present study is the infrequency of such interaction in some courts. Apparently, in some courts there is rarely a report or testimony by a mental health professional, even on issues in which such opinions are thought to be *de rigeur* and even dispositive.[2] Frankly, we are puzzled by this finding, which deserves further study.

Because there is little relationship between presentation of such reports and community size, it is unlikely a matter of accessibility to mental health professionals (cf. Melton, 1983a) And given that judicial attitudes toward the use of mental health professionals were not consistently related to the frequency of such testimony and reports in their courts, the lack of such opinions is unlikely to be simply a matter of judicial caprice. It is possible that the prosecution in some jurisdictions commonly stipulates incompetence or insanity when there is a serious question about a defendant's mental state. Another possibility, also unverifiable by our data, is that the judges who indicated that they seldom hear a report or testimony by a mental health professional even in cases of civil commitment and competency to stand trial routinely receive only the clinician's conclusion by phone or letter (hence, no report or testimony). Regardless of whether this hypothesis is accurate or whether there is actually no involvement in the mental health system, the implication is that defendants often have no real access to the expert development of evidence pertaining to their mental state.

1. A recurring problem in mental health law has been the misidentification of such issues as being medical rather than legal and moral (Morse, 1978). The result has been that clinical opinions are often dispositive, especially in competency to stand trial (Roesch & Golding, 1980) and civil commitment proceedings (*see, e.g.,* Hiday, 1977, 1981; Stier & Stoebe, 1979; Warren, 1977). Judges have a preference for clinicians' giving ultimate-issue opinions even in matters of criminal responsibility; they also prefer theoretical, diagnostic opinions over the presentation of "hard" research data (Poythress, 1982b).

2. *See supra* note 1.

This conclusion is rendered still more disturbing by the fact that much of the information about mental health that judges do receive often occurs through occasional self-initiated consultation with behavioral-science experts or literature. For most judges, this consultation is sufficiently irregular that they are unlikely to have a full appreciation of a psychological issue. The danger then is of a judicial notice being made from an incomplete or inaccurate understanding of a given psychological phenomenon without the parties in a case having an opportunity to rebut the judge's conclusions (Perry & Melton, 1984; Saks & Baron, 1980).

Our concern is an ambivalent one, however. *Some* knowledge is probably better than no knowledge, and judicial colleges and informal consultation may often be the easily available means of sensitization to psychological issues. Perhaps the best means, though, is ongoing, rather than sporadic, mental health consultation to courts. The data in the present study suggest that typical training experiences of judges do not affect their attitudes toward or knowledge of forensic mental health.[3] It is useful, therefore, to examine both sides of the potential interaction. What is the nature of the involvement of community mental health professionals with the legal system?

Mental Health Professionals and the Courts

METHOD

Participants. In summer 1981, the forensic teams in the *E* clinics and in the various comparison groups (i.e., clinicians in the *E* clinics who were not members of the forensic teams, master's- and doctoral-level clinicians in the *C* clinics) were administered a questionnaire about the frequency of their interaction with the legal system at the same time they took the test of forensic knowledge (results are reported in chapter 3). Only persons who had been actively involved in community mental health were included. Thus, for example, psychology residents at the University of Virginia were omitted from the sample for this study. The total sample size was 147, including the members of the forensic teams in the *E* clinics.

Procedure. Participants were asked to identify their discipline, level of education, primary job function (i.e., direct clinical service delivery, consultation and

3. We do not mean to imply that continuing education is intrinsically ineffective. Focused training with respect, for example, to models of forensic service delivery might result in more reasoned referrals.

education services, supervision and training or staff development, administration), and extent of formal forensic training (i.e., current demonstration program, previous training programs at the Institute of Law, Psychiatry and Public Policy, other continuing education workshops, coursework during graduate school or residency program). They also indicated the frequency of their personal involvement in referrals for services from each of the following persons or agencies: juvenile and domestic relations court (judge or court service/probation staff); district and circuit courts (judges or court service/probation staff); commonwealth's attorney; defense attorney; local jail or detention center (sheriff's office).

The participants were then asked the frequency of their personal involvement in each of various services to the legal system: evaluation of competency to stand trial or mental state at the time of the offense; jail crisis intervention, including prescreening of prisoners for civil commitment; dispositional or pre-sentence evaluation; treatment, including treatment as a condition of probation or of dismissal of charges; program-related consultation or mental health education; case-related consultation (other than simply sending an evaluation or treatment report). Finally, the participants estimated the frequency of their contact with a professional from the legal system by each of the following means: telephone call; letter, memo, or report; face-to-face contact in court; face-to-face contact outside court.

Blank responses were omitted from statistical analyses. For some analyses, adjacent cells were combined to eliminate cell frequencies that were too small to perform a chi-square test.

RESULTS

Frequency of Involvement. Most community mental health professionals apparently have infrequent involvement in referrals from the legal system, especially from attorneys (see Table 15). About three-fifths of the sample reported that they are involved in referrals from defense attorneys no more than twice a year, and even more (about four-fifths) reported such sparse involvement in referrals from prosecutors. Community clinicians tend to be involved with court-ordered treatment. Although a substantial proportion of clinicians (40.8%) rarely have even this involvement, forensic treatment is much more common than forensic evaluation or consultation. The form of the interaction is generally impersonal; face-to-face contact with a legal professional outside court happens fewer than three times a year for two-thirds of the sample, and even less frequently (for about three-fourths of the sample) inside court. However, almost two-fifths of the sample reported that they have phone conversations with legal professionals more than once a month.

Table 15: Frequency of Community Mental Health
Professionals' Contacts with the Legal System

Referral Source	Never	1 to 2 Times a Year	Once a Month or Less	1 to 4 Times a Month	More Than Once a Week
Juvenile and domestic relations court	24 (16.3%)	36 (24.5%)	58 (39.5%)	22 (15.0%)	7 (4.8%)
District and circuit courts	25 (17.1%)	39 (26.7%)	49 (33.6%)	19 (13.0%)	14 (9.6%)
Commonwealth's attorney	64 (43.5%)	53 (36.1%)	16 (10.9%)	10 (6.8%)	4 (9.5%)
Defense attorney	35 (23.8%)	56 (38.1%)	32 (21.8%)	18 (12.2%)	6 (4.1%)
Local jail or detention center	35 (23.9%)	42 (28.8%)	35 (24.0%)	26 (17.8%)	8 (5.5%)
Service Provided					
Evaluation of competency to stand trial or mental state at time of offense	90 (61.6%)	21 (14.4%)	14 (9.6%)	15 (10.3%)	6 (4.1%)
Jail crisis intervention	62 (42.2%)	45 (30.6%)	17 (11.6%)	18 (12.2%)	5 (3.4%)
Presentence evaluation	65 (44.2%)	34 (23.1%)	36 (24.5%)	9 (6.1%)	3 (2.0%)
Treatment	21 (14.3%)	39 (26.5%)	54 (36.7%)	20 (13.6%)	13 (8.8%)
Program-related consultation	67 (45.6%)	36 (24.5%)	22 (15.0%)	9 (6.1%)	13 (8.8%)
Case-related consultation	42 (28.5%)	49 (33.3%)	32 (21.8%)	12 (8.2%)	11 (7.5%)
Form of Contact					
Telephone call	6 (4.1%)	23 (15.6%)	61 (41.5%)	39 (26.5%)	18 (12.2%)
Letter, memo, or report	13 (8.8%)	37 (25.2%)	60 (40.8%)	23 (19.0%)	9 (6.1%)
Face-to-face in court	59 (40.4%)	53 (36.3%)	20 (13.7%)	11 (7.5%)	3 (2.1%)
Face-to-face outside court	39 (26.5%)	54 (36.7%)	34 (23.1%)	15 (10.2%)	5 (3.4%)

Note: $N = 147$; some n's equal less than 147 because of blank responses.

Factors Affecting Frequency of Interaction. Although the questionnaire was filled out only a few months after completion of training and before the pilot project was fully implemented in some *E* jurisdictions, members of the forensic teams were significantly more likely than the *C* clinicians to have involvement with the legal system for all referral agents, all functions except treatment, and all forms of interaction except phone calls (see Table 16). It is noteworthy that this relatively high level of involvement was true even for some functions (e.g., jail crisis intervention) which were not a focus of the pilot project. However, having had other forms of training in forensic mental health (e.g., continuing education workshops, coursework in graduate school) did not relate significantly to frequency of involvement with the legal system.

It is also noteworthy that even the forensic teams often did not venture inside the courtroom, at least in the early stages of the pilot project's development. Only 15.4 percent of the trainees reported in-courtroom interaction with legal professionals more than once a month, and 26.9 percent said that they never have such interaction. Face-to-face interaction outside court was relatively common, however. Almost one-third of the trainees had such involvement more than once a month.

Area of professional discipline was also related to the frequency of involvement. Psychiatrists were more likely to have extreme levels of involvement with legal professionals (i.e., frequent interaction or no interaction at all) (see Table 17). These disciplinary differences were apparently not simply a result of differential assignment of the clinics' most highly trained staff. Comparisons of doctoral (M.D., Ph.D., D.S.W., and Ed.D.) and subdoctoral staff showed significant differences only for frequency of interaction with juvenile courts, $\chi^2 (3) = 13.41$, $p < .01$, and commonwealth's attorneys, $\chi^2 (3) = 8.12$, $p < .05$, and in both cases these differences were substantially smaller than the corresponding disciplinary differences.

Position at the clinic was remarkably unrelated to frequency of interaction with legal authorities. Staff whose primary function was reported as administrative or supervisory were more likely than staff whose primary duties are in service delivery to participate in program-related consultation with legal professionals, $\chi^2(3) = 9.19, p < .05$. Most of this difference was accounted for by staff who reported that they *never* performed such consultation (51.8% of clinical staff and 24.2% of administrative/supervisory staff). There was also a marginally significant difference between clinical and administrative/supervisory staff in frequency of forensic treatment, $\chi^2(3) = 6.42, p < .10$. Otherwise, there were no significant differences on the basis of position in the frequency of interaction with the legal system, with respect to any of the variables studied.

DISCUSSION

Two general findings stand out. First, community mental health clinics typically have minimal involvement in the legal system. When they do, it tends to be as a resource for court-ordered treatment, most likely as a condition of probation or a plea bargain. Second, the pilot project substantially extended the involvement of clinics in the legal system, including functions other than evaluations in criminal cases.

The low level of involvement that community clinics have in the legal system

Table 16: Relationship between Forensic Training
and Frequency of Contacts with the Legal System

Referral Source	Never	Once a Month or Less	More Than Once a Month
Juvenile and domestic relations court**			
Pilot project	1	16	9
Other forensic training	7	9	1
No forensic training	26	71	16
District and circuit courts			
Pilot project	0	9	17
Other forensic training	5	9	3
No forensic training	20	69	13
Commonwealth's attorney***			
Pilot project	1	14	11
Other forensic training	8	8	1
No forensic training	54	47	2
Defense attorney***			
Pilot project	1	12	13
Other forensic training	7	6	4
No forensic training	27	69	7
Local jail or detention center***			
Pilot project	1	10	14
Other forensic training	4	8	5
No forensic training	30	68	15
Evaluation of competency to stand trial or mental state at the time of the offense***			
Pilot project	2	7	17
Other forensic training	13	3	1
No forensic training	75	24	3
Jail crisis intervention**			
Pilot project	3	14	9
Other forensic training	8	8	1
No forensic training	50	40	13
Presentence evaluation**			
Pilot project	4	16	6
Other forensic training	8	8	1
No forensic training	52	46	5

Table 16: *continued*

Referral Source	Never	Once a Month or Less	More Than Once a Month
Treatment			
Pilot project	4	18	4
Other forensic training	2	12	3
No forensic training	15	63	25
Program-related consultation***			
Pilot project	3	16	7
Other forensic training	11	5	1
No forensic training	52	37	14
Case-related consultation***			
Pilot project	1	14	11
Other forensic training	6	9	2
No forensic training	35	57	10
Phone call			
Pilot project	1	16	9
Other forensic training	2	7	8
No forensic training	4	71	28
Letter, memo, or report***			
Pilot project	1	7	18
Other forensic training	1	10	6
No forensic training	11	79	13
Face-to-face in court			
Pilot project	7	15	4
Other forensic training	8	7	2
No forensic training	44	50	8
Face-to-face outside court*			
Pilot project	2	16	8
Other forensic training	4	10	3
No forensic training	33	61	9

Note: $N = 147$; some n's equal less than 147 because of blank responses. All tests for statistical significance are based on $\chi^2(4)$ analysis.
*$p < .05$ **$p < .01$ ***$p < .001$

may reflect a general retrenchment in services. Several studies (e.g., Woy, Wasserman, & Weiner-Pomerantz, 1981) have noted the tendency for clinics to move away from consultation and education as their federal staffing grants expired. Centers then depended almost exclusively on traditional clinical services for generating fees. The federal Mental Health Systems Act included a provi-

84

Table 17: Disciplinary Differences in Frequency of Contact with the Legal System

Referral Source	Never	Once a Month or Less	More Than Once a Month
Juvenile and domestic relations court***			
Medicine/psychiatry	8	4	4
Nursing	0	4	2
Counseling	2	14	4
Psychology	8	31	13
Social work	5	41	5
District and circuit courts*			
Medicine/psychiatry	5	5	6
Nursing	1	5	0
Counseling	3	10	7
Psychology	7	35	10
Social work	7	33	10
Commonwealth's attorney**			
Medicine/psychiatry	8	3	5
Nursing	5	1	0
Counseling	5	13	2
Psychology	18	29	5
Social work	27	22	2
Defense attorney**			
Medicine/psychiatry	6	4	6
Nursing	4	2	0
Counseling	4	14	2
Psychology	8	35	9
Social work	11	33	7
Local jail or detention center*			
Medicine/psychiatry	5	4	7
Nursing	1	4	1
Counseling	5	11	4
Psychology	8	34	9
Social work	15	24	12

Note: $N = 147$; n's equal less than 147 because of blank responses. All tests of statistical significance involved $\chi^2(2)$ analyses, comparing physicians with nonphysicians.
*$p < .05$ **$p < .01$ ***$p < .001$

sion, repealed before it was implemented, that would have provided grants specifically earmarked for services that are not revenue producing.[4] These financial disincentives for community involvement have coincided with the growing belief among many mental health professionals that the fervor for social change which guided the early community mental health movement was naive and misplaced (see, e.g., Group for the Advancement of Psychiatry, 1983).

Also, something about the legal system may deter involvement by community mental health centers. The legal system's case-by-case focus on narrow issues (cf. Davidson & Saul, 1982) and its different jargon and world view (see Melton et al., in press, chap. 1) may make it unattractive to centers that maintain a community orientation. The clients of the legal system, especially in criminal law, may also be perceived as more "bad" than "mad" and unfit for mental health intervention.

Finally, the restrictions that the legal system itself places on mental health professionals' input may make it difficult for community clinics to provide forensic services. The extreme levels of psychiatrists' involvement are noteworthy in that regard. The disproportionate number of psychiatrists who never consult to the legal system probably reflects a more individualistic, medical-model orientation than the other mental health professions. Practical considerations are probably also important, however. As money has tightened, there has been a steady decline in the number of psychiatrists in community centers (see Group for the Advancement of Psychiatry, 1983; Langsley & Barter, 1983), and the limited amount of psychiatric time available is often earmarked for prescribing and monitoring medications and supervising clinicians of other disciplines.[5] At the same time, however, the legal system has persisted in a preference for *medical* testimony in many jurisdictions (Dix & Poythress, 1981).[6] The disproportionate number of psychiatrists with a high level of involvement in the legal system may be a result of this preference. The practical reality then is that an inefficient

---

4. 42 U.S.C. § 9435 (Supp. IV 1980). The grants programs under the Mental Health Systems Act were repealed and replaced by the Alcohol and Drug Abuse and Mental Health Services Block Grant, 42 U.S.C. §§ 300x-1 *et seq.* (Supp. V 1981).

5. This narrow use of psychiatrists' time is especially likely when, as was the case in Virginia, medical supervision is required for reimbursement by third-party payers. This practice was held to be an illegal monopolistic policy in Blue Shield of Va. v. Va. Acad. of Clinical Psychologists, 450 U.S. 916 (1981).

6. Va. had such a preference for physicians' testimony, although clinical psychologists were permitted to testify to at least some issues, *see* Rollins v. Commonwealth, 207 Va. 575, 580-81, 151 S.E.2d 622, 625-26, *cert. denied*, 386 U.S. 1026 (1967). The statute enacted in Virginia subsequent to the pilot project (see appendix E) provides clearly for qualification of psychiatrists and clinical psychologists. A recommendation that master's-level psychologists and social workers also be permitted to testify as to competency to stand trial (Commissioner's Committee, 1982) was rejected by the General Assembly.

distribution of staff resources may be necessary for community mental health centers to provide forensic services in jurisdictions that do not recognize psychologists and social workers as being mental health experts.

Conclusion: Toward a Community-Oriented, Community-Based Forensic Service System

The studies reported in this chapter are only a beginning. The study of community mental health centers is limited to a single state, and the sample of judges is national but not fully representative. Both studies rely on self-report with its accompanying distortions. The present studies need to be followed with research in other jurisdictions and by other methods (e.g., archival data). In particular, it would be useful to learn more about why some courts frequently hear opinions from mental health experts and why other courts rarely do. Also, further study is needed about the determinants of interdisciplinary attitudes of both judges and mental health professionals.

Nonetheless, the data from the two studies fit sufficiently well with each other and with our experience (see chapter 6) that we feel confident in drawing some general conclusions. Apart from systematic incentives (such as the commissioner-level directives in the Virginia pilot project), courts and community mental health centers rarely interact. Indeed, many judges seldom have direct encounters with the behavioral sciences either in or out of court, and even more community mental health professionals are rarely in contact with legal professionals.

This situation is unfortunate in our view. The lack of adequate forensic services in the community is likely to affect adversely the quality of justice in individual cases (see chapter 1). More broadly, the legal system is a primary mechanism for channeling interpersonal disputes in our society, and it is unfortunate that community mental health centers have been isolated from it. Although it would be a mistake to conceptualize the legal system as a giant therapy center, formal links between the legal system and the centers might be useful additions to consultation programs at the centers. Attorneys may benefit from consultation on interviewing and counseling skills. Formal links with the legal system may also facilitate outreach to persons in distress who otherwise might not seek mental health services. Ongoing consultation with court officials might also stimulate more effective and humane practices. The early involvement of many of the Virginia forensic teams in jail crisis intervention is noteworthy in that regard (cf. Runck, 1983). Consultation might result, for example, in more rational policies with respect to diversion from the criminal justice and civil commitment systems.

Although the establishment of community-based forensic services is a worthy goal in itself, the ultimate goal should be the development of *community-oriented,* community-based services. Consultation that stops with the interview of a defendant and the provision of a report is unlikely to provide substantial help to an attorney who is trying to defend a "difficult" client. More generally, it also stops short of the potential use of clinic-court links to benefit a larger segment of the community. Community-based forensic services should be seen then in the larger context of community mental health ideology.[7] They offer greater possibility for justice in individual cases in which mental disorder is at issue, but community-based forensic teams also may have many opportunities for significant program-related consultation.

7. The Mental Health Systems Act (which is now repealed, *see supra* note 4) expressly required community mental health centers to provide consultation to courts and law enforcement and correctional agencies, 42 U.S.C. § 9411(b)(1)(A)(iv)(I) (Supp. IV 1980).

Chapter 6

Problems of Program Implementation

This chapter describes the Virginia pilot project, its by-products, and the lessons we learned from the experience of planning for, establishing, and monitoring the program described in the preceding chapters. As such it is in large part impressionistic and contains subjective evaluations of the actors involved and the political and social factors that played a role in the project. The first three sections of the chapter divide the experience into three historical periods: before, during, and after the pilot project. The final section attempts to summarize the most salient lessons drawn from the experience.

Laying the Groundwork for the Pilot Project

The idea for establishing a system of community-based outpatient forensic evaluations in Virginia came from a number of different sources. The state Department of Mental Health and Mental Retardation, the University of Virginia's Institute of Law, Psychiatry and Public Policy, and various individual lawyers and mental health professionals were pushing for such a system as early as 1976. Each group had its own reasons for advocating outpatient evaluations, but they all shared at least two concerns about the hospital-based evaluation system in existence at the time: One, the cost of hospitalizing defendants ($100 a day for over seven hundred defendants a year) and transporting them to and from the hospitals amounted to well over $1.5 million a year. Two, pretrial hospitalization of defendants lasted an average of thirty days, which appeared to be much longer than necessary for most evaluations and therefore was in violation of defendants' constitutional rights to bail, least restrictive treatment, and speedy trial. Of course, for both of these points we assume that many who were hospitalized did not need to be. The first objective, then, was to generate information on this issue.

In conjunction with the department, the institute sponsored a preliminary study that examined the records of all defendants hospitalized for forensic evaluation in 1976 (McCall, 1979). The results of this study indicated that perhaps 70 percent of the defendants who were committed to Virginia's hospitals for criminal reasons did not require prolonged inpatient observation or treatment. These data, combined with evidence from other states such as Tennessee, Massachusetts, Ohio, and Missouri indicating that community-based systems could work (see chapter 1), allowed us to ask the state legislature for funds to set up a "test" training program (to be distinguished from the later pilot project, which not only trained mental health professionals but also set up a system in which they could operate). The department's request for funding this test program was granted in 1977, and the training began at the institute's facilities in 1978.[1]

Even with the department's encouragement, it was hard to attract mental health professionals to an eight-day program which, because evaluations were still hospital-based, could not promise that the knowledge it imparted would be useful. Most of the clinicians who participated in the training sessions were from clinics located close to the institute's facilities. Others could not afford the cost of travel. Fortunately, however, by 1979 enough trial runs of the training had taken place to make it possible for the institute to recommend to the department that a full-fledged pilot project be established. As earlier chapters of this book describe, the project was to be a way of testing an evaluation system in which community professionals would provide front-line evaluation services on an outpatient basis. The department was fully in favor of the proposed project, especially because one of its two maximum-security hospitals, Southwestern State, was to be turned over to the Department of Corrections, leaving only one hospital available to perform forensic evaluations.

1. At this point, it might be useful to say something about the relationship between the institute and the department. The institute, which consists of personnel from the law and medical schools at the University of Virginia, is only partially supported by the university. The grant from the department thus was a welcome source of income. The department, on the other hand, was looking for, and found in the institute, a source of expertise in the area of mental health law. With its staff of lawyers, psychiatrists, psychologists, and social workers and its contacts with the professional and academic groups these individuals represented, the institute is a rich resource. The department was able to take advantage of the institute's know-how at a cost probably no greater and perhaps less than what it would have paid had it tried to develop this capacity internally (the average contract between the department and the institute was $100,000 a year once the pilot project was fully underway). The nature of this collaborative effort is illustrated by the test training program. The institute could offer the practical and scholarly insight necessary to run a competent effort, but it was the department's money and contacts that made the program possible.

This symbiotic relationship continues. In fact, the relationship may be too successful. The attorney general's office has recently demanded that the institute's contract with the department clearly indicate that all policy formulations by the institute be funneled through the attorney general's office before presentation to the commissioner of the department. This move undoubtedly was triggered by the intimate connections that institute personnel have developed with department staff.

Thus, in January 1980, a proposal and request for funds for the two-year study was submitted to the legislature. The only real opposition came from a powerful prosecutor in the state who feared that graduates of a program run by the University of Virginia might be more likely than the hospital staff to find people insane or to recommend "soft" dispositions. Such resistance from the prosecutor lobby would become a recurring problem (discussed later in this chapter). However, it did not prevent the Virginia General Assembly from agreeing with the department's proposal, and on March 8, 1980, the legislature passed House Joint Resolution No. 22 (see appendix B), which had been drafted by staff of the department, the attorney general's office, and the institute. As described in chapter 2, the resolution called for the Department of Mental Health and Mental Retardation to establish a Forensic Evaluation Training and Research Center and further directed the commissioner to help the center set up "demonstration services projects" in selected jurisdictions. With the authorization that H.J.R. 22 provided, the pilot project was ready to begin.

The Pilot Project: Establishing and Defending the Program

The research that took place during the pilot project is described in earlier chapters of this book. This section discusses the practical difficulties encountered in trying to implement a demonstration system for outpatient forensic evaluations. It is helpful to look at the implementation process in terms of four different initiatives undertaken by the center, specifically, (a) arranging for the court system to pay the community mental health professionals trained by the center for each evaluation; (b) selecting and training mental health professionals from the six target communities; (c) educating members of the bench and bar in the target jurisdictions about the pilot project; and (d) monitoring the progress of the project by providing, as needed, continuing education of and consultation with the trainees. We discuss each of these areas at length.

COMPENSATION
Under the original proposal for the pilot project, evaluations performed in the community were to be financed by the department. Thus, H.J.R. 22 specifically stated that the "demonstration service projects" were to provide evaluations for the courts "without fee," meaning that they would be reimbursed through appropriate adjustments in their funding from the department. Yet the General Assembly, either intentionally or through a bureaucratic slipup, did not appropri-

ate the money to the department to pay for these evaluations. Thus, the first job of the center was to find a source of funding for the evaluations.

For several months, it appeared that the legislature's oversight would be the demise of the program. Without compensation, community professionals were unlikely to participate in the project, as the institute's experience during the test training made clear. Although several sources of money were considered, the most logical seemed the court system, because judges, lawyers, and probation officers are responsible for requesting most forensic evaluations. Moreover, Virginia law already provided that private clinicians who performed evaluations for the courts were entitled to up to $200 per evaluation and report.[2] The problem was that under this statute reimbursement varied from judge to judge and frequently was not forthcoming.

Thus, in July 1980, the center approached the executive secretary of the Supreme Court of Virginia, whose office supervised disbursal of state court funds, in an effort to guarantee fiscal stability for the pilot project's evaluations. Negotiations with the executive secretary's office were prolonged; the primary sticking point, of course, was why the courts should assume a cost that the Department of Mental Health and Retardation, via its hospitals, had always shouldered. The center argued, ultimately successfully, that (a) the department's primary obligation was to treat, not evaluate; in fact, were it not for the courts, the department would not be involved in evaluation capacity at all; (b) the new system should improve the quality and efficiency of the evaluations requested by the courts; (c) if the courts did not pay for the evaluations, the quality of evaluations would suffer, because of the imminent shutdown of Southwestern State; (d) the project should reduce the *overall* state budget because it would decrease expenditures at the hospitals by a sum greater than the expenditures of the courts; and (e) the project was experimental in any event; the wisdom of the payment system could be reassessed in two years.

The executive secretary's office was also concerned that the center's proposal involved paying for sentencing evaluations as well as evaluations for competency and mental state at the time of the offense (MSO). Under the statute, it was not clear whether the $200 limitation was per evaluation or per individual. With the help of the attorney general's office, which construed the statute broadly to encompass all evaluations at $200 per evaluation, these concerns were overcome.

Eventually, a document was drafted that provided $100 for each combined competency and MSO screening evaluation (see chapter 1 for a description of

2. Va. Code § 19.2-175 (1975).

the latter assessment), $200 for each comprehensive MSO evaluation, $200 for a presentence evaluation if no prior psychological evaluation had been performed in the case, and $100 for presentence evaluations in cases where previous evaluations had taken place. A recent version of this document, which now governs all outpatient evaluations in the state, is found in appendix F. In drafting this so-called memorandum, we were careful to explain why the new compensation system was necessary, the rationale for outpatient evaluations generally, and the fact that the department, the executive secretary, and the attorney general's office were fully behind the concept of outpatient evaluations.

Even with the guarantee of compensation from the courts, many problems arose. Some judges did not pay attention to the new fee schedule; others quibbled over how it was to be interpreted. Moreover, there was a significant lag between the time evaluations were performed and payment was received. With the exception of the latter problem, these difficulties disappeared as the system adjusted, and the reimbursement hiatus was not a major irritant once payments began coming in, because they were then continuous, although six months to a year behind schedule.

SELECTION AND TRAINING OF MENTAL HEALTH PROFESSIONALS
With the memorandum on compensation signed, the center had little trouble convincing clinics to send clinicians to the training. Of the several clinics initially approached about the project, only two balked. Both were in suburban areas with relatively well-off clientele and a small criminal court caseload; both stated that they could not spare the staff for the project and that the evaluations would not pay for themselves. Conversely, the remaining clinics saw the program as a potential money-maker because so many of the other services they provided to the community were performed gratis. Many also felt that the evaluations were an integral part of what a community clinic should be doing.

The center focused on clinics, rather than private clinicians, partly to facilitate its research, but also because it felt that clinics were much more likely than often-transient, individual clinicians to be able to develop an ongoing relationship with the court system. After the pilot project research was completed, however, private clinicians who requested the training were accepted if they paid a small tuition fee.

In approaching the clinics, the center told each clinic director that participation in the project would involve sending, at the clinic's expense, a team of three to five professionals to a training program at the center's facilities in Charlottesville. Given Virginia's expert qualification requirements, this team would have to include one psychiatrist or doctoral-level clinical psychologist. The clinic would also be asked to provide various types of data to the center once evaluations began. In exchange, the staff would be certified to perform forensic evaluations reimburseable at the rates set out in the reimbursement memorandum. These demands on the clinics would create some difficulties for later participants in the program. Fortunately, the six original target clinics were all able to send psychiatrists or doctoral-level psychologists to the pilot training as well as a sufficient number of other staff.

The training of the clinicians from the target clinics was completed by March 1981. The complete course continues to be six days of instruction at the center plus one day of supervised evaluation at Central State Hospital in Petersburg. The topics covered at the center and the length of time spent on each are as follows: the legal system—sources of law and legal procedures (2 hours); the application of the fifth amendment to the forensic process (1 hour); the imprecision of the behavioral sciences—implications for the forensic specialist (1 hour); competency to stand trial—legal and clinical considerations (6 hours); evaluation of mental state at the time of the offense—the screening evaluation (2 hours); supervised competency and screening evaluations (6 hours); comprehensive evaluations—information gathering, psychological testing, and interview technique (3 hours); sentencing—legal considerations (1 hour); amenability to treatment and dangerousness evaluations (2 hours); juvenile courts—legal and clinical considerations (3 hours); report writing (1 hour); expert testimony and consultation with the courts (3 hours).[3]

Each trainee also received a 350-page training manual containing outlines and relevant background materials. Those who attended this course and passed an eighty-question forensic evaluation (discussed in detail in chapter 3) received a certificate indicating that they had completed the forensic training program given at Virginia's Forensic Evaluation Training and Research Center.

We will not describe here the paradigmatic confrontations encountered in teaching one discipline about another (see Melton et al., in press, chap. 1), except to say that probably the biggest pedagogical problem was getting across to the trainees the narrow focus and unique purpose of a forensic evaluation. As forensic specialists, their job would be assessment, not therapy or disposition; and their primary obligation would be to the court, not the patient. Regarding technique (as opposed to substance), we found that lectures were probably necessary to lay the groundwork, but substantial use of illustrative videotapes and involvement of the trainees in performing and critiquing evaluations were extremely effective.

After each course (the six target clinics were trained in two groups of three),

3. The materials developed on these subjects eventually evolved into a book dealing comprehensively with forensic evaluation (Melton et al., in press).

we asked for evaluations of the training and received very high marks. Feedback from the trainees, once they began evaluations, turned up one area in which the training was deficient: practical hints on how to set up contacts with the various members of the legal system and to maintain good relations with them. We now endeavor to add such information whenever possible. For instance, trainees are instructed that it is extremely important for each clinic to have a single phone number where members of the evaluation team can be reached, that clinicians evaluating defendants in the jail need to make arrangements for a suitable interview room, and that formal feedback sessions with members of the legal system would enhance communication.

Ultimately, however, it became clear to us that regardless of how well we prepared the clinicians, the success of any relationship with the legal profession depended on lawyers' understanding what the clinicians had to offer. Thus, the next phase of the project marked the beginning of perhaps the most important part of the center's efforts at establishing an outpatient evaluation system.

EDUCATION OF THE BAR

In January and February of 1981, after training was completed but before the trainees began performing evaluations for the courts, meetings were held in each target jurisdiction. Judges, prosecutors, and defense attorneys were invited. Clerks, sheriffs, and jail personnel were also encouraged to attend, because they would play an integral part in the project (clerks often process orders and set evaluation dates; sheriffs transport defendants to be evaluated outside jail; jail personnel arrange interviews; all are valuable sources of background information). Of course, the trainees were also present.

Each meeting followed the same format. Those who attended (unfortunately, often less than a third of those invited came) received a twenty-page booklet containing H.J.R. 22, the reimbursement memorandum from the Supreme Court, and model court orders and reports. After everyone was introduced, members of the center, often accompanied by a representative from the attorney general's office, explained how the program was expected to operate and then answered questions.

The questions and comments during these sessions revealed a number of different concerns about the pilot project. Probably the most common complaint about the proposed system was its prohibition on ultimate-issue language in the reports submitted by the clinicians. Ultimate-issue language expresses an opinion on a legal issue using the words of the test devised to analyze that issue. Judges and lawyers had for years received conclusory, one-paragraph letters from the hospital evaluators using such language on competency and sanity issues (e.g., "the defendant is competent," "the defendant is insane," or "the defendant knew right from wrong at the time of the offense") and had come to appreciate the straightforward answers these reports contained. Although recognizing that Virginia law on the subject is far from clear,[4] many of the lawyers (especially judges and prosecutors) at the jurisdictional meetings insisted that the clinicians in the project continue the practice of using legal terminology in delivering their opinion on the defendant's competency to stand trial and mental state at the time of the offense. This preference from judges and lawyers has been noted elsewhere (Poythress, 1982a; Morse, 1982c). Some judges also stated that they did not want lengthy reports that included detailed supporting information. They said such reports were confusing or could contain irrelevant information, which the defendant would not want revealed.

Members of the center and the trainees tried to explain their belief—and that of virtually all scholarly commentators on the issue (e.g., American Psychiatric Association, 1982; Bazelon, 1982; Bonnie & Slobogin, 1980; Goldstein, 1967; Morse, 1978; Task Force on the Role of Psychology in the Criminal Justice System, 1978)—that clinicians possessed no expertise to address legal issues and instead should provide judges and lawyers with the raw data and clinical inferences from those data, which would be relevant to those issues (see Morse, 1978). Experts should *assist,* not displace, the fact finder. These debates often reached an impasse. In one meeting, two judges stated that they would continue to use the hospitals until the center's policy on the use of legal language was changed.

These exchanges highlighted the tenuous position the center occupied midst academic idealism, practical reality, and the official lawmakers of Virginia. Many subjects taught in the training program (e.g., clinical use of legal terminology, the application of the fifth and sixth amendments to forensic evaluations, see Slobogin, 1982, and the "diminished-capacity" doctrine)[5] had not been addressed or only superficially considered by the Virginia legislature, judiciary, and attorney general's office. Yet the center felt that definitive stances needed to be taken on these subjects, either because the program would not work well otherwise (as with the fifth amendment issue) or because scholarship and the law in other states strongly supported them, as with the ultimate-issue and diminished-capacity ideas (Arenella, 1976; Dix, 1971). As the center found,

4. No Virginia case deals with the issue in the context of mental health law. Several hold, in civil cases, that the witness may not address an ultimate issue of fact to be decided by the jury. *See, e.g.,* Oliphant v. Snyder & Gunter Oil Corp., 147 S.E.2d 122 (Va. 1966); Grasty v. Tanner, 146 S.E.2d 254 (Va. 1966); Venable v. Stockner, 108 S.E.2d 380 (Va. 1959).

5. The phrase "diminished-capacity doctrine" is meant to refer to the use of clinical testimony on the issue of whether the defendant possessed the cognitive mental state, or mens rea, for the offense charged. It is to be distinguished from expert testimony on insanity, which focuses on the affective and volitional, as well as the cognitive, impairment of the individual at the time of the offense.

attempting to establish a workable program and at the same time to introduce novel and unappealing concepts to many members of the bar created considerable difficulties.

Although the controversy over what language clinicians should use in their reports and testimony created some opposition to the program among individual judges and lawyers, the two subjects that stimulated the most-heated and best-organized response to the pilot project were the application of the fifth amendment to the evaluation process and the diminished-capacity concept. Following what it believed to be the legally correct (if not constitutionally required) approach (Slobogin, 1982), the center had told the trainees not to include any offense-related information in reports sent to the prosecution until after the defendant had given formal notice that he or she wished to raise a psychiatric defense. In addition, the center had explained the notion that clinical testimony might be admitted not only on the issue of insanity but also on the question of whether the defendant possessed the requisite mental state for the offense.[6] These two positions caused a vigorous reaction from the prosecutor "lobby" and nearly destroyed the credibility, if not the viability, of the pilot project.

The prosecutors felt that they should be able to request an evaluation of the defendant's competency *or* insanity any time after arrest. Virginia law at the time did not provide authority to order insanity evaluations; the only statute relevant to forensic assessment dealt solely with competency evaluations.[7] But for years lawyers and judges had been able to obtain any type of evaluation they wanted, whenever they wanted it. The prosecutors also argued that it was their duty as officers of the court to seek evaluation and hospitalization of a defendant who might be insane. From this they concluded that they should be able to obtain the results of any evaluation reports, regardless of whether they contained incriminating information or whether the defendant intended to rely on them at trial. Pointing out that wealthy defendants were able to take advantage of the attorney-client privilege to protect prenotice evaluation results and that indigent defendants were thus unfairly prejudiced did not sway the prosecutors.

The fact that the center taught the trainees about the diminished-capacity

6. Over half the states have permitted such testimony, finding it unconstitutional to deny the defendant relevant evidence, *see, e.g.,* Commonwealth v. Walzack, 360 A.2d 392 (Pa. 1976). But many others have refused to admit it on one or more of the following ground(s): (1) that evidence of mental abnormality is admissible only on the issue of insanity; (2) that permitting such evidence might lead to complete acquittal (as opposed to commitment after an insanity acquittal); (3) that expert evidence on mens rea is unlikely to be based on specialized knowledge.

7. Va. Code § 19.2-169 (1975).

doctrine reinforced some prosecutors' earlier impressions (discussed in the previous section) that the center was too liberal to be entrusted with training community professionals. The one case in Virginia relevant to the issue is equivocal.[8] The prosecutors therefore concluded that the subject should not be taught. The center felt that since clinicians were in fact often permitted to testify about mens rea (criminal intent) in Virginia courts, they should be prepared to do so competently.

So far the criticisms of the pilot project involved interpretation of legal principles. A second set of complaints resulted from what might be called misperceptions about the nature of forensic clinical evaluations. Criticism of the first type could be countered through persuasive "teaching" of legal concepts. Criticism of the second type required an even more laborious education process, because when it came to clinical matters, lawyers possessed little or no knowledge.

The most vehement reaction of the second type challenged the very premise of the pilot project. Several judges and lawyers felt that outpatient evaluations would not work, that "good" assessments of competency and insanity required days, weeks, and even months of observation. The center staff stressed that the efficacy of outpatient evaluations was exactly what was being assessed in the pilot project and that previous research and experience (reviewed in chapter 1) had suggested that such evaluations were feasible (Roesch & Golding, 1980; Stone, 1975). But many of the legal professionals did not put much stock in this research. They regarded it as counterintuitive: evaluations had always been performed in the hospital, and the idea that an evaluation of legal insanity and an assessment of "what's wrong" with a person are one and the same thing.

Legal professionals are socialized to think in terms of deference to precedent. Although such a style is illogical when it is used to test the truth of a factual proposition (as opposed to the validity of a legal conclusion), it is often applied to such decisions (Perry & Melton, 1984). Thus, any reform in the legal system is likely initially to be viewed by lawyers and judges as illegitimate to the degree that it departs from the way things have always been done. Similarly, the medical model embedded in mental health law (see Melton et al., in press, chap. 1) may lead judges to infer that the hospital is necessarily the place for forensic evaluations and treatment.

A second and related reaction was distrust of the screening concept for mental state at the time of the offense. Lawyers did not believe such a short evaluation was possible, and, even if it was, it would often be misleading. At the time, the results of our study suggesting the reliability of the screening device (see

8. Dejarnette v. Commonwealth, 74 Va. 867 (1881).

98

chapter 1) were not available; instead, we pointed out that most defendants did not have a valid psychiatric defense and that the screening evaluation should therefore vastly improve systemic efficiency. A third concern, often raised by sheriffs, was whether an outpatient system would provide sufficient security. Our response was that most evaluations would be performed in jail, but even those that were performed at the clinics should not present significant security risks if the ten-year experience at the institute's own forensic psychiatry clinic was any guide.

A final "clinical" issue that created discomfort among members of the legal profession was the project's reliance on psychologists and social workers as well as psychiatrists to perform evaluations. Many were not convinced that persons other than psychiatrists were competent to conduct forensic examination; others felt that even if they were, their credibility as experts could not compare with that of a psychiatrist and that they would therefore be of small aid to lawyers whose opposition had retained one (but see Petrella & Poythress, 1983). We cited case law qualifying psychologists to perform evaluations of mental state at the time of the offense[9] and social workers to perform competency evaluations[10] and pointed out that the team approach advocated by the project should result in reports that are more carefully thought-out and balanced (see Dix & Poythress, 1981).

Most of these misperceptions about clinical expertise did not disappear during the meetings held at the target jurisdictions. Nor did the disputes over the correct legal postures for the project. One prosecutor sent a letter to the commissioner of the department, with copies to the center and ten other prosecutors in the state, complaining that a report submitted by one of the trainees had addressed treatment issues (which he implied was an inappropriate attempt to influence the judge in the defendant's favor rather than an effort to address the defendant's restorability to competency). Another politically powerful prosecutor told the commissioner about his grave concern over the pilot project and his hope that the "situation" would soon be corrected. In an effort to defuse some of the tension, the center's staff met twice with a committee of prosecutors, but the meetings were inconclusive.

Finally, in May 1981, the center and the department established an advisory committee consisting of seven judges, five defense attorneys, and six prosecutors. Its mission was to advise the center on the conduct of the pilot project.

9. See, e.g., Simmons v. Mullen, 331 A.2d 892 (N.J. 1974); Hogan v. State, 496 S.W.2d 594 (Tex. 1973); People v. Davis, 62 Cal. 791, 402 P.2d 142 (1965).
10. See, e.g., People v. Parney, 253 N.W.2d 698 (Mich. 1977), which suggests that under some circumstances social workers may testify on competency issues. Tennessee qualifies social workers and other types of mental health professionals by statute. See Tenn. Code Ann. § 33-708 (1976).

Had this committee been set up soon after the passage of H.J.R. 22, much of the controversy surrounding the program may have been avoided. Because of its politically diverse nature, the committee provided a forum in which the center could present its side without feeling defensive and which considered all points of view. Indeed, after its first meeting, the committee agreed that (a) the information in the clinics' reports should be used only to address the issue of the defendants' mental condition; (b) the diminished-capacity doctrine should be taught in the training program; (c) outpatient evaluations and screening evaluations were good ideas and feasible (based on the committee's own assessment of the ongoing program and on the center's preliminary data for the first three months of the project); and (d) Ph.D. clinical psychologists should be given statutory authority to perform any type of forensic evaluation.

The one area where the committee and the center parted ways was on the use of legal language by clinicians. The committee agreed unanimously that mental health professionals should be able to use ultimate-issue terminology in their reports. Most committee members expressed a desire that such language be *required* in every report, although it was suggested that evaluators clearly label their conclusion as an opinion or recommendation. As a result of this decision, the center advised the trainees to end each of their competency reports with the following language: "It is our opinion that, according to our interpretation of the legal standard in [the section of the Virginia Code defining competency] the defendant is (in)competent to stand trial." However, the center continued to advise its trainees to avoid using the words *sanity* or *insanity* in their reports, unless expressly directed to do so by the courts. This compromise rested on the belief that the gap between clinical opinion and legal conclusion is relatively easily bridged in competency determinations but would require too great a leap into murky moral questions about insanity.

As this experience suggests, the committee's opinions were advisory only. But those opinions which favored the center's position did stall the movement against the pilot project by providing an official expression of support and co-opting the prosecutors who sat on the committee, which included as members some of the most voluble critics of the project.

An added advantage of the committee (and probably the most appropriate function of such a group) was that it provided, through a formal mechanism, a means of obtaining legal expertise on problems associated with the pilot project. For example, its members helped draft model court orders and suggested useful changes in the content of the training program.

Thus, the advisory committee improved the image of the project and assisted it in tangible ways as well. Other attempts to educate the bar—for instance, speeches at the annual meetings of Virginia's district court judges and the Commonwealth's Attorneys Association—probably also had a positive effect. Undoubtedly, the best rebuttal of complaints about the project came from the operation of the project itself. Many of these complaints disappeared in the face of the program's success and the communication between disciplines that developed because of it.

Solid evidence that suspicions about the program had begun to dissipate once it was underway was provided by a survey conducted fifteen months after the pilot project began. In June 1982, we sent a questionnaire to all district, circuit, and juvenile court judges in the six target jurisdictions, as well as the commonwealth's attorneys and three defense attorneys in each jurisdiction. A detailed description of the survey and its results is found in chapter 4. Here, briefly, we point out that in five of the six target jurisdictions, there was consistent agreement among the three groups of legal professionals that the quality of services provided by the clinics was high. In the remaining jurisdiction, only two of the seven respondents rated the clinic poorly. Moreover, because both respondents gratuitously signed their names to their responses, the center was able to identify them as the two judges who had threatened to continue using the hospitals if the project did not change its policy regarding conclusory language.

The results of the survey were gratifying. But it was clear from talks with members of the legal community that the project needed a firmer foundation than the goodwill of the lawyers who made use of it. The center's attempts to obtain legislation explicitly supporting its viewpoints is described in the latter section of this chapter.

CONTINUING EDUCATION AND MONITORING

Throughout the pilot project, the center's staff stayed in close contact with the trainees, advising them of developments on the political front, keeping them abreast of changes in the law and forensic advances, and monitoring their progress. This communication was accomplished through a variety of mechanisms. About once a month, the center sent out a newsletter describing important events of the past weeks and enclosing, when necessary, supplements to the loose-leaf training manual. Over the phone, the center provided consultation on specific problems and kept track of the project's day-to-day operation. The staff also visited each clinic at least twice between March 1981 and March 1982 to discuss how the program was working. One of the more valuable aspects of these visits was the opportunity to observe the trainees perform evaluations in their own environment. The clinics were also asked to provide random samples of their evaluation reports, which were reviewed and critiqued by the center's staff. (The report evaluation study, described in chapter 4, was conducted wholly independently of this critique, which was designed for educational rather than research purposes.)

The center also engaged in formal continuing education programs. Each clinic team spent one day at Central State performing evaluations with the outpatient evaluation protocols developed by the center. And in November 1981 and May 1982, the center sponsored forensic symposia in Charlottesville. During these gatherings, to which all the trainees were invited, center staff apprised the group of new developments (such as the Supreme Court's decision in *Estelle v. Smith*)[11] and provided additional training, assisted by members of Central State's staff. These symposia would become a semiannual fixture of Virginia's evaluation system and a valuable method of exchanging information.

On June 30, 1982, the pilot project officially came to an end. The two years of the project provided considerable insight into the practical problems of initiating a system heavily dependent on interdisciplinary cooperation and understanding. It also provided time for the center to develop a clear idea of priorities for the outpatient evaluation system. The center continues to implement those priorities.

Consolidating the Gains after the Pilot Project

Well before the pilot project ended, the staff of the Forensic Evaluation Training and Research Center became involved in several activities that fell outside the literal mandate of H.J.R. 22. Yet each of them was designed to assure that the project would have a chance of surviving and expanding once this mandate expired.

The first such activity in which the center became involved was planning for and implementing a statewide outpatient evaluation system. The drafters of H.J.R. 22 contemplated taking this step only after the final report of the pilot project had been received by the Department of Mental Health and Mental Retardation, sometime in the summer of 1982. However, several developments led the department to begin planning and setting up such a system much earlier than originally anticipated. Most significantly, the previously mentioned shutdown of the forensic unit at Southwestern State Hospital and an overall increase in demand for evaluations had begun to put substantial strain on the staff at Central State Hospital (Commissioner's Committee on Mental Health and Mental Retardation Services, 1982).

11. 451 U.S. 454 (1981).

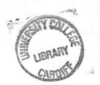

Bolstered by preliminary research findings from the project indicating that the target clinics were reducing hospital admissions, members of the department, Central State, and the center met in July 1981 to discuss how the system should be structured. It was decided that the center would immediately begin training for additional community clinics (avoiding the control clinics involved in the pilot research). In the meantime, to meet the demand for forensic services during the time required to train these clinics, clinicians from the six civil hospitals were to attend the training program. As noted in chapter 4, these clinicians, once trained, began performing outpatient forensic evaluations, *at the hospitals,* of defendants from jurisdictions that did not yet have trained staff in clinics. For jurisdictions with trained clinicians, the hospitals would function as backup evaluation facilities.

Eventually, the core concept of providing outpatient evaluations at both the clinic and hospital levels became official department policy under commissioner Joseph Bevilacqua. As described in the Final Report of the Commissioner's Committee on Mental Health and Mental Retardation Forensic Services,[12] issued in April 1982, the system would consist of a "graduated three-tiered statewide system for conducting forensic evaluations using community-based resources (Level I), regional civil hospitals (Level II), and the Central State Hospital Forensic Unit (Level III)," as well as "a graduated statewide system for conducting *inpatient* forensic evaluation using regional civil hospitals, at least one designated medium security forensic unit, and Central State Hospital Forensic Unit." The report also suggested that a central forensic office be established within the department to oversee and coordinate the three tiers. Under this system, which continues in operation, the hospitals perform evaluations only when no community service exists, when an inpatient evaluation is necessary, or, occasionally, when the court system wants a second evaluation. Central State's services are generally reserved solely for inpatient evaluations of extremely dangerous patients or for those requiring special expertise, as in capital cases.[13]

In the early days of planning for and setting up this system, the members of Central State Hospital—since the July 1981 closing of Southwestern State— became the only hospital-based forensic experts and manifested an ambivalent attitude toward the center and the community evaluation program. On one

12. Three members of the institute staff, Richard Bonnie, John Monahan, and Christopher Slobogin, served on the committee that produced this report.
13. It should be noted, however, that some judges in jurisdictions located near one of the four state hospitals tended to avoid the clinics and send defendants needing evaluation directly to the hospitals. Virginia's director of forensic services is therefore considering a prohibition of outpatient hospital evaluations of any defendants from jurisdictions which have clinics available.

hand, they wanted some relief from the burden of performing most of Virginia's forensic evaluations. On the other, they naturally enjoyed their status as the sole "experienced" forensic clinicians in the state and were not entirely sure, again quite naturally, that community professionals were "up to snuff." Moreover, much of the content of the training program (in which they too participated) implicitly criticized their way of doing things (e.g., conclusory reports). Central State's support of the community program was important, because its staff was respected by the legal community, especially by the prosecutors. Yet throughout 1981, some members of the staff expressed qualms about the pilot project. Only gradually did they throw their support behind the program, perhaps partly because of the center's efforts to make use of their expertise and experience in the training program and the forensic symposia, and perhaps partly because they became convinced of the project's efficacy. They may also have realized that, whatever their feelings about the matter, the department was fully committed to the concept of outpatient evaluations. Today the ambivalence seems to have disappeared. The hospital staff and the center have a strong relationship with the common objective of improving evaluation services in Virginia. Indicative of this relationship was the hospital's cooperation in several of the studies reported here.

Paralleling its efforts to restructure the evaluation system in Virginia, the center began a concerted push to rewrite Virginia law on the subject of forensic evaluations, to provide firm authorization for the type of evaluation system the pilot project represented. As noted earlier, the only statute relevant to the issue focused on competency evaluations. It was phrased in ambiguous and archaic language and failed to incorporate several new developments in constitutional law. In May 1981, partly as a result of the center's efforts, the secretary of human resources commissioned a task force to suggest revisions of this statute. Two members of the center were appointed to the task force and were instrumental in drafting a new version.

On March 1, 1982, the Virginia General Assembly passed the draft with only a few modifications, and it became effective July 1, 1982.[14] The new statute requires the courts to use outpatient evaluation services whenever they are available, provides that certain background information be forwarded to the evaluators before they begin their evaluation, fully protects the fifth-amendment rights of those evaluated, requires the judge to consider ordering outpatient treatment for defendants who are found incompetent to stand trial or are in need of emergency treatment, and authorizes psychologists, as well as psychiatrists, to perform evaluations of competency and mental state at the time of the of-

14. Va. Code §§ 19.2-169.1 to 19.2-169.7 (1975).

fense (see appendix E). The statute thus gave the outpatient evaluation system a firm legal footing and boosted implementation of the plan.

Coincident with the statute's passage, the office of the executive secretary of the Supreme Court of Virginia promulgated model court orders, prepared with the assistance of the center, incorporating the requirements of the new law (see appendix G). Perhaps more than the statute, the order forms and the instructions accompanying them help promote the outpatient evaluation concept because they are used every day by those who run the criminal justice system. Also as a result of the new statute's passage, the executive secretary's office agreed to sign a new reimbursement memorandum extending the fixed-fee schedule described earlier to evaluations performed by *any* clinic with staff trained by the center (see appendix H).

Finally, as a result of its experience with the state's computer system during the pilot project, the center became involved in advising the department and the Supreme Court on the proper coding of information concerning forensic evaluation and treatment. Without accurate and easily accessible data, policy decisions can be based only on educated guesses.

At the present time the center's main function is to train a new group of mental health professionals every two months. Clinicians from almost two-thirds of Virginia's clinics and from all of the major hospitals have been trained. Conducting the training in Charlottesville, rather than where the clinics are located, presents financial problems for some clinics, which as a result may not send as many clinicians to the training. Similarly, not all clinics can afford to send a psychiatrist or Ph.D. clinical psychologist to Charlottesville for a six-day program. Taking the training on the road, however, will probably not occur until the demand for it subsides. Moreover, presenting certain parts of the program (e.g., live evaluations, videotape vignettes) would not be possible in some locations.

The Lessons Learned

The following presents a summary of suggestions about how to plan for, establish, and operate an outpatient evaluation system. We have developed a list of do's and don'ts for implementing the type of program described in this book.

1. *Involve all key actors in both the mental health sector and the legal system at the initial planning stages.* Although the Department of Mental Health and Mental Retardation, the attorney general's office, and the institute worked closely

together from the beginning, other institutions and groups did not become involved until much later in the program. This was a mistake. Political controversy and turf battles could have been avoided or minimized had all the relevant groups been solicited for input from the outset. From our experience, the groups that should be consulted are several:

(a) *The mental health department.* Any effort to establish an outpatient evaluation system without support from the agency which is responsible for evaluating and treating criminal defendants would be futile. Indeed, the primary impetus for initiating such a system will presumably need to come from this agency. The agency will be able to use its links with community clinics, other governmental agencies (such as the attorney general's office and the court system), and the legislature to encourage participation in and support for the system. Virginia's Department of Mental Health and Mental Retardation enthusiastically backed the pilot project and has appointed a director of forensic services who oversees the community evaluation system as well as evaluation and treatment in the hospitals.[15] This central coordination within one office is probably the most efficient method of administering the system.

(b) *The attorney general's office.* A number of legal issues arise in establishing an outpatient evaluation system. During the pilot project, they ranged from the correct interpretation of the reimbursement statute to the appropriate stance on the diminished-capacity issue. The attorney general's office can give opinions on these issues which, if supportive of the program, can be helpful in persuading lawyers in the criminal justice system to endorse the program's objectives. Virginia's attorney general's office was active in construing current statutes, in a way that fortunately bolstered the aims of the project. On the other hand, it remained aloof during the battles over the content of the training program. As it turned out, this aloofness probably benefited the project.

(c) *Hospital staff.* Individuals who perform evaluations at the hospitals have connections throughout the system and can provide valuable expertise on clinical and legal issues. They can also be useful resources in identifying key actors in the relevant systems and various interjurisdictional idiosyncracies. Such information can be very helpful in project implementation. Moreover, because the nature of their jobs will be affected by the initiation of an outpatient evaluation system (i.e., fewer evaluations, more treatment), hospital staff should be kept informed of all program developments. As noted earlier, one mistake the center made was not taking advantage of Central State's experience in performing forensic evaluations and not involving the hospital's staff in early planning sessions.

15. Joel Dvoskin was the director at the time of the study.

(d) *Representatives from the legal system.* As the experience with the prosecutors and the advisory committee suggests, it is absolutely crucial to develop a relationship with prosecutors, judges, and defense attorneys at the earliest possible stage of planning. Valuable advice and useful support can be obtained from well-known, knowledgeable individuals in each of these three groups. The inherent conservatism of the legal system can be overcome to some extent through direct involvement of key members of the bench and bar who are educated about the advantages of the system and can communicate these advantages to their colleagues.

(e) *The agency responsible for court administration.* If the plan is to reimburse the clinics through the courts, the need for this liaison is self-evident. Additionally, this agency is responsible for drafting and disseminating model court orders and directing judges on the practical aspects of court administration. Finally, this agency is usually responsible for training judges. For all of these reasons it was necessary for the center to develop a good working relationship with the Supreme Court's executive secretary's office at an early date.

(f) *Directors of community clinics.* These individuals must be supportive of the outpatient evaluation idea in order for it to work. The costs and benefits of the program should be explained to each of them. In return, the directors can offer suggestions on the content of the training, the logistics of reimbursement, and the best way to deal with members of the bar in their own community. Attracting clinics was not overly difficult. Although the Department of Mental Health and Mental Retardation had some leverage over Virginia's clinics (in the form of various disbursements connected with state grants), it did not coerce them into participating; the center was able to "sell" the idea of a community-based program to virtually all clinics. Even those that were originally reluctant to get involved have joined the program. Probably the biggest selling point is the flat-fee reimbursement schedule negotiated with the Supreme Court.

(g) *A university affiliation.* Although probably not critical to the project's success, the association between the Department of Mental Health and Mental Retardation and the University of Virginia, which the center represented, ensured a quality program that will keep up-to-date on both legal and clinical developments. The university affiliation also provides a mechanism for ongoing evaluation research and a base that is relatively free of the direct political influences, which could distort the objectivity of forensic services.

A university association is not without its drawbacks, however. In particular, the project's connection with the so-called liberal University of Virginia may have damaged its credibility with some prosecutors and judges.

2. *Obtain legal authorization.* The passage of H.J.R. 22 was probably the single most important event of the pilot project. This document proved to members of

the mental health and legal communities that the project was legitimate and that it had the full backing of the legislature. Without this document, the center would have had a much more difficult time convincing lawyers that they should make use of the new services rather than continue to use the hospitals.

Similarly, as noted, the reimbursement memorandum made it possible for the center to assure naturally cautious clinics that compensation for evaluations was forthcoming and to convince judges that they were obligated to authorize flat-fee payment when evaluation reports were received. If the project had had to depend on judicial interpretation of the preexisting compensation statute (cited earlier), the clinics and the courts might not have participated in the project as fully as they did.

Interestingly, neither H.J.R. 22 nor the reimbursement memorandum was a statute or regulation. A resolution is merely a means of expressing the "sense of the legislature" on a particular issue, and the memorandum, although signed by the commissioner and a representative of the attorney general's office, was not produced through the promulgation process normally required for a valid regulation (e.g., public hearings with notice).

Ideally, of course, before a program of this nature is contemplated, a state would enact a statute that, like the current Virginia law, requires outpatient evaluations when outpatient services are available and that settles many of the legal questions the center had to wrestle with during the two years of the pilot project. Although such a statute could not have been passed before the pilot project began (after all, the purpose of the project was to ascertain whether an outpatient evaluation system was feasible), it now is on the books in Virginia, and research supports the approach it calls for. Such support may make it easier to pass similar statutes in other states.

Finally, as noted earlier in this chapter, one of the important accomplishments with respect to the everyday workings of the new system was the promulgation of model court orders geared to the statute. Such forms assist the busy judge in conforming to the dictates of a statute that he or she may not have had time to read carefully and helps lawyers and clinicians sort out their roles.

3. *Develop training materials for the community clinicians which reflect, as much as possible, a consensus view of the law.* Any attempt to arrive at the "correct" view of the law in areas that have not been definitively ruled on will be difficult. This problem is exacerbated by judges, prosecutors, defense attorneys, and the attorney general's office who naturally have their own views about these subjects and because none or only some of these views coincide with the approach advocated by the "commentators." Thus, a consensus view on, for example, the correct application of the fifth amendment to psychiatric evaluations, the ultimate-issue issue or the definition of "mental disease or de-

fect" for purposes of the insanity defense is not possible, unless statutory or case law has succinctly decided these issues.

There is an obvious relationship between the first two lessons discussed in this section and this one. To the extent that an advisory committee, the attorney general, or the state legislature *can* arrive at fully informed uniform conclusions about such issues, the training entity is relieved of the burden of deciding what to teach. Because we did not have such assistance on most issues, we were forced to devise our own approach and consequently walked into controversy that could have been at least partially avoided through diligent preproject communication with the appropriate parties. Had the center been able to invoke the imprimatur of, for instance, the advisory committee on the legal and clinical issues that stirred reaction among the legal community, the path toward a working system probably would have been smoother.

Of course, one danger of seeking such an imprimatur is that the content of the training may be dictated by a group which is not fully informed about the issues. Moreover, some members of the bench and bar will always doubt the wisdom of certain practices or teachings regardless of the support for them. For example, as noted earlier, many lawyers were not particularly impressed with research about the efficacy of outpatient evaluations performed in other states, even after the advisory committee came out in support of the concept. This was particularly true of lawyers who knew of "a case" in which the defendant's "true nature" was not revealed until after several days or weeks of observation. The "representativeness" heuristic (see Saks & Kidd, 1980) was frequently encountered by members of the center.

There are two ways of dealing with this problem. One is to compromise on some issues, in particular those which appear to be the most important to the legal profession. Otherwise, the program may fail because of bullheaded allegiance to an approach which may be philosophically correct but which, in the overall scheme of things, is not of enough significance to cause the sacrifice of the entire project. The center's compromises on the ultimate-issue question and the issue of whether social workers are qualified to perform competency evaluations are two examples of such compromise.

Of course, one can compromise too much. Therefore, the second, and better, approach to dealing with difficulties in reaching a consensus with members of the bar is to persuade them of the benefits of the approach advocated, which leads to the next observation.

4. *Arrange for formal training of legal professionals which emphasizes the fiscal and systemic benefits.* The center not only held jurisdiction-by-jurisdiction meetings, but also participated in annual gatherings of prosecutors, the defense bar, and judges and now occupies a permanent slot on the agenda of the an-

nual training program for district court judges. Efforts to seek contacts beyond these sessions are encumbered because the bar does not see mental health issues as having that much relative significance, a perception which is probably accurate in view of the pervasive problems associated with our criminal justice system. And in the meetings the center participated in, attempts to educate the bar about the benefits of an outpatient evaluation system were often less than successful, at least at the outset.

Two factors furthered the education process as the pilot project matured. One was the daily contact between members of the legal profession and the mental health profession; this contact helped convince skeptics that the system could work and that not every defendant would be found insane by the newly trained evaluators. The second factor was the completion of research which tended to show that an outpatient system would save the state money. Unlike other types of research, these data seemed to impress legislators, judges, and lawyers alike. This is not to say that concerns about the defendants' constitutional rights or the quality of evaluation services were not relevant to these groups. However, it is clear that the hard numbers showing reduced costs tended to receive more attention than arguments or research related to substantive philosophical and legal concerns, whether the forum was negotiations with the Supreme Court over reimbursement, testimony in the state legislature in favor of the new statute, or speeches to the Commonwealth's Attorneys Association. In a very real sense, the success of the project depended on its ability to relieve the state budget. This capacity provided a point of alliance with groups that might not have been philosophically attuned with a least-restrictive-alternative approach.

Bottomline money issues also proved important to the community clinics. We have already noted that clinics' participation was typically based on projected fees as well as ideology. These concerns have persisted. Thus, some participating clinics have tended to refer screened-in defendants to Central State Hospital for comprehensive evaluations of mental state at the time of the offense. Screening evaluations are perceived as fiscally profitable, but comprehensive evaluations are not.

5. *Seek continuous feedback from all sectors.* An obvious corollary of seeking input from all relevant groups at the initial stage of the project is to continue to solicit suggestions and comments throughout the program. Through conferences, phone calls, and newsletters, the center was able to keep apprised of developments within each jurisdiction and to refine its own approach to various problems. Observations of the first two years of the pilot project suggested new legislation in the principal areas requiring firm statutory guidance.

Other problems discovered as a result of feedback were not susceptible to legislative solution because they arose only in certain jurisdictions and were better handled through informal methods. For instance, courts in many urban areas had already developed contacts with mental health professionals in private practice who were willing to perform evaluations at the community level; in these areas, there was less acceptance of the new program relying on clinics and nonpsychiatrists. After obtaining feedback from the first experiences dealing with this situation, however, the center and the department became adept at incorporating preexisting connections between the courts and the clinical community into the outpatient evaluation system. Over time, many of the private clinicians were coaxed into attending the training program and developing formal or informal relationships with the center.

As these examples illustrate, the most important benefit of feedback is the opportunity it provides to keep the system responsive to the diverse and often idiosyncratic needs of each jurisdiction and at the same time to ensure that any "variances" from hoped-for or stated objectives do not stray too far. As Reppucci and Saunders (1983) have demonstrated, a coherent philosophy is necessary but not sufficient to achieve systemic change. Equal attention must be given to historical context, staff attitudes, decision-making structure, and political conflicts, if a program is to be fully implemented. Without continuous monitoring and sensible modification of the program, the overriding objective of an outpatient evaluation system—the efficient provision of quality evaluation services—will not be met.

Chapter 7

Toward a Model System of Forensic
Services: Recommendations for Policy

To return full circle to the point we introduced at the beginning of this volume, attention needs to be given to the *procedures* as well as to the standards for the introduction of expert assistance by mental health professionals into the legal system. Such a focus on the process of law and mental health interaction is necessary to ensure that (a) the quality of input is high, (b) defendants' rights are protected, (c) forensic services are delivered in a cost-effective manner, and (d) the integrity of the mental health professions is protected.

In chapter 1, we reviewed the evidence suggesting that these goals are most likely to be met in a community-based system of forensic services. However, we also noted that there had been no comprehensive evaluation of such a system. Consequently, the argument for a community-based system was essentially hypothetical, albeit based on analogous and consistent empirical findings.

A comprehensive evaluation was necessary to ensure that the projected quality and cost-effectiveness of a community-based system would in fact be achieved without undesirable side effects. For example, there was the pos-sibility of a net-widening effect whereby the same defendants would still be sent to an inpatient maximum-security facility, but with an unnecessary additional step of having a community-based evaluation. Alternatively, the existence of easily accessible forensic services might sufficiently increase the number of referrals to obliterate any cost savings, or the services in the community might supplement rather than replace hospital-based services. As discussed in chap-ter 1, sketchy data from Tennessee and Ohio suggested that these net-widen-ing effects might in fact occur. Tennessee saw an increase in referrals for foren-sic evaluation after community mental health centers began offering this service, and the initial Ohio community centers emphasized presentence eval-uations and probation-related treatment, services which had not been provided by Lima State Hospital. Moreover, similar experiences had been reported in other attempts to use community-based treatment programs (e.g., juvenile di-version programs) to divert offenders from institutional correctional facilities (see, e.g., Nejelski, 1976). A net-widening effect is not per se undesirable. If defendants *needing* services were not receiving them, justice would demand the expansion of the clientele of the forensic mental health system. However,

the high proportion of defendants ultimately found competent, for example, suggested that the forensic mental health system is more likely to be abused
through overuse.

The decision by the Virginia General Assembly to initiate a demonstration
program of community-based forensic services[1] provided an opportunity to perform the evaluation research necessary to assess the actual functioning of such
a system. The General Assembly's unusual express directive for evaluation
research on the pilot project[2] established the authority to test the hypotheses
about the superiority of a community-based system in a close approximation of
a true experiment. Thus, the Virginia project offered a relatively clear test of the
efficacy of community-based forensic services, with the possibility of minimally
equivocal conclusions and, therefore, sound empirical bases for policy.

Conclusions

The major findings reviewed in this volume may be summarized as follows:

1. The opportunity for rampant abuse of the forensic mental health system
exists particularly when services are provided on an inpatient basis (chapter 1).
Among the potential costs to defendants are deprivation of the constitutional
rights to bail and a speedy trial and de facto punishment without due process.

2. A carefully designed community-based forensic evaluation system results
in a substantial reduction in inpatient admissions and a corresponding reduction
in fiscal costs (chapter 2).

3. A net-widening effect is not an inherent result of a community-based system; admissions may in fact be reduced by proportionately greater amounts
over time, as the system becomes more established (chapter 2).

4. There is in fact a core of specialized knowledge in forensic mental health
that is unlikely to be shared by either general clinicians or legal fact finders
(chapter 3).

5. It is possible to educate general clinicians in this body of knowledge in
several days of workshops (chapter 3).

6. This training improves the quality of reports of forensic evaluations, as
rated by trial judges, prosecutors, and defense attorneys (chapter 4).

7. Community mental health centers typically have minimal interaction with

1. House Joint Resolution No. 22 (1980).

2. *Id.,* requiring the Forensic Evaluation Training and Research Center established by the resolution "to compile the necessary information for evaluating the success of this [community-based forensic services] program" (purpose 4).

the legal system (chapter 5). Analogously, in some jurisdictions courts seldom have input by mental health professionals even in cases where such consultation is often thought to be standard.

8. Designation of community mental health centers as the source of criminal forensic evaluations may have the side effect of increasing interaction between the mental health center and legal authorities on other issues (chapter 5).

9. Successful implementation of community-based forensic services requires much more than simply training community mental health clinicians in the techniques of forensic assessment (chapter 6). Notably, the system can fall apart without active involvement—or without co-optation—of all the relevant parties (e.g., state mental health and court administrators, judges, prosecutors, defense attorneys, sheriffs, directors of community mental health centers, guild organizations of the various mental health professions).

10. Many of the legal issues that are inevitably raised in determining the scope of, and procedures for, forensic evaluation are not settled, "black-letter" legal matters. The development of forensic services can be stymied by a lack of sensitivity to these issues and the various positions on them (chapter 6).

In short, the studies in the Virginia project, taken in sum, confirmed the predictions derived from previous research that community-based forensic services can be of high quality and substantially less expensive than inpatient services. In view of the significantly reduced infringement on defendants' rights in community-based services, these studies give ample support for development of predominantly community-based systems of forensic services. In chapter 6, we examined the process of implementation of such a system and provided the rudiments of a "how-to" manual for development of community-based forensic services. In the remainder of this chapter, we offer recommendations for policies governing the design of forensic services.

Recommendations for Policy

ORGANIZATION OF SERVICES

Recommendation 1. Forensic services should be delivered in the least restrictive alternative. As discussed in chapter 1, it is a basic principle of constitutional law that infringement on constitutionally protected interests should be no more intrusive than necessary to meet compelling state purposes.[3] Given that most forensic evaluations and at least some forensic treatment can be per-

3. *See* Shelton v. Tucker, 364 U.S. 479, 488 (1960).

formed on an outpatient basis, deference to the least-drastic-means principle requires a presumption in favor of community-based services (see ABA, 1983, Std. 7-4.3 and commentary). A corollary to this guideline is that *there should be a multi-tier approach to forensic services.*

Evaluations should generally be performed on an outpatient basis, although there may be rare cases in which more extensive observations or special procedures (e.g., sodium amytal interviews) are desired which can be best performed within a hospital.[4] Often forensic treatment services can be performed on an outpatient basis (see, e.g., ABA, 1983, Std. 7-4.9[a] and commentary). In that regard, in some jurisdictions defendants who enter the mental health system for the purpose of treatment are often not accused of violent offenses.[5] Thus, unless treatment requires inpatient care, public safety is unlikely to require hospitalization of such defendants. Treatment needs can also be met in the community. For example, a mentally retarded defendant found incompetent to stand trial can be best "restored" to competency through focused special educational services that can be delivered most effectively in the community because it is easier to work with the defendant's attorney and to familiarize the defendant with the courtroom there. Similarly, an acutely psychotic defendant may sometimes be restored to competency with phenothiazines and other treatments (e.g., day hospital) delivered on an outpatient basis.

In some cases, however, the least restrictive alternative is some form of inpatient treatment. This conclusion does *not* mean, though, that in such cases the least restrictive alternative will necessarily be maximum-security treatment (ABA, 1983, Std. 7-7.6 and commentary). Thus, there is a need for intermediate-level services. This need is frequently present even for insanity acquittees who are confined for continuing dangerousness. As they improve, increasingly less restrictive alternatives are likely to be possible and desirable steps toward reintegration into the community.

An intermediate level of services may also be necessary for evaluation when the case is particularly complicated or requires extended observation. There may be some cases, for example, in which certain evaluation questions can only be answered through treatment or in which there is substantial risk of decompensation when the defendant is forced to recall events at the time of the offense.

---

4. A need for hospitalization for forensic evaluation does not necessarily translate into a need for hospitalization in a special forensic hospital, even in these rare instances.

5. Among the jurisdictions in which substantial numbers of insanity acquittees are charged with nonviolent offenses are Missouri (Petrila, 1982) and Oregon (Rogers & Bloom, 1982). Moreover, although a disproportionate number of defendants found incompetent to stand trial are charged with serious offenses, the most common charges against incompetent defendants are serious property crimes (see, for review, Roesch & Golding, 1980, pp. 52–54).

Recommendation 2. Whenever possible, forensic services should be inte-grated with regular mental health services. We have several reasons for prefer-ring to minimize separation of forensic services in special centers or hospitals. First, such an integration is consistent with prevailing trends in mental health. The community mental health movement is based in part on a premise that psychological interventions should be available in, and directed toward, the so-cial systems in which people actually experience stress. Second, and related to the first point, much of the work of a well-functioning forensic services system may be thought of as consultation, a primary means of promoting community mental health. As noted in chapter 1, the competency evaluation by its very nature seems to demand consultation with the defense attorney in techniques of communication with a difficult client. Similarly, it is obviously true that many people in distress seek help through the legal system. Thus, community mental health centers have an opportunity to reach these persons indirectly through consultation with legal authorities. Programs of mental health consultation to police and neighborhood justice centers indicate a possible expansion of foren-sic services to preventive mental health services in the legal system (cf. Melton, 1983a). Third, integration of forensic services into the regular mental health system minimizes the possibility of their becoming de facto correctional ser-vices. Fourth, such integration also minimizes the possibility of forensic ser-vices being the unwanted stepchild of the mental health system, chronically underfunded and understaffed. Fifth, legitimacy of forensic services in the men-tal health system is likely to promote the recruitment and retention of skilled forensic clinicians in the public sector.

The last three reasons are really hypotheses, albeit testable ones, which are based on the experience of isolated forensic services and are consonant with intuition. We are reasonably confident in these predictions, but they should be directly tested in future research.

In the meantime, our recommendations for services which are delivered in the least restrictive alternative and integrated with the regular mental health system lead to a conclusion that most forensic services should be provided by community mental health centers. We are aware, however, of the arguments of some mental health administrators (e.g., Petrila, 1981) that a preferable means of decentralization of forensic services is to locate them in regional hospitals. Less administrative coordination would be required. And the proponents of the regional-hospital model make two principal assertions about the practicality of the model of the community mental health centers. First, in rural areas there may be insufficient numbers of mental health professionals with the credentials necessary to gain acceptance in court as experts. Second, in some commu-nities there may be insufficient numbers of cases to give clinicians the neces-sary experience in forensic assessment to achieve desensitization of the notion of talking with rapists and murderers and to learn the nuances of work in the legal system. The latter reason is not persuasive because practical experiences can be incorporated into forensic training. The former reason may have merit, given the prevailing shortages of psychiatrists (Langsley & Robinowitz, 1979) and doctoral-level clinical psychologists (Richards & Gottfredson, 1978) in many rural areas.[6]

In any case, we have no serious quarrel in principle with the regional-hospital model, *provided* that forensic evaluations and, whenever possible, forensic treatment are delivered there on an outpatient basis. Nonetheless, we are still convinced that the community-based model is optimal. As already noted, community-based forensic services are consistent with the philosophy of community mental health and their functions of consultation and education. Moreover, state hospitals are less likely than other mental health settings to be able to attract qualified staff (Morse, 1982a; Stone, 1982).

Recommendation 3. The forensic service system should be comprehensive. When possible, each tier of the system should be prepared to offer the full range of forensic services. Without such capability, abuse of the system is more likely. Less restrictive settings may seek an "out" to have undesirable (e.g., unprofitable) services provided outside the community,[7] and attorneys, too, may attempt to use the ruse of unavailability of a particular service as a means of hospitalizing the defendant for illegitimate reasons (e.g., delay, detention without bail). Also, if particular forensic services are unavailable, attorneys and judges may couch referral questions in terms of the services provided (e.g., competency evaluation) instead of what is really desired (e.g., emergency treatment, consultation on management of the defendant in jail, development of information useful in plea bargaining; see Hastings & Bonnie, 1981; Roesch & Golding, 1978, 1980). The result is often the unnecessary and costly provision of a particular service that does not adequately fulfill the actual perceived need.

Recommendation 4. In the design of the forensic service system, careful attention should be given to the protection of defendants' rights. This recommendation underlies this entire discussion, as exemplified by the emphasis on ser-

6. The argument that rural communities are unlikely to have the professionals necessary for a forensic team may have less merit than appears on first glance. Many rural community mental health centers are in fact *regional* rather than *community* in scope. Ozarin (1982) has pointed out that some rural catchment areas exceed 50,000 square miles.

7. Apparently some centers in the Virginia system have been performing screening evaluations but then referring defendants for full evaluations to Central State Hospital because the comprehensive evaluations are perceived as requiring too much staff time for the level of reimbursement available.

vices in the least restrictive alternative. However, we are reiterating the point for two reasons. First, it has been our experience that these fundamental justifications for community-based forensic services tend to get lost in consideration of economic benefits. Indeed, as noted in chapters 2 and 6, bottomline concerns persuaded Virginia authorities of the merits of community-based forensic services. The substantive reasons for such a system attracted much less attention. Second, some of the constitutional issues with respect to the design of forensic services are subtle, complex, and frequently neglected. For example, as briefly discussed in chapter 6, the application of the fifth and sixth amendments to forensic evaluations is a matter of considerable controversy as well as substantial significance for the preservation of defendants' interests in an adversary system (for more extensive discussion, see Melton et al., in press, chap. 3; Slobogin, 1982).[8] Less subtly, many states have failed to adopt procedures consistent with the strictures of *Jackson* for release of incompetent, unrestorable defendants (Steadman & Hartstone, 1983; Winick, 1983).[9]

One implication of these observations is that it is important to include lawyers knowledgeable about both mental health law and forensic assessment in the design and implementation of forensic services. Mental health clinicians and administrators understandably are more likely to be concerned with, and knowledgeable about, the psychological rather than the legal aspects of forensic assessment, despite the ethical injunction at least for psychologists to "avoid any action that will violate or diminish the legal and civil rights of clients or others who may be affected by their actions" (American Psychological Association, 1981, Principle 3c).

A second implication is that procedures designed to protect defendants' rights in the forensic services system should be spelled out in statutes (preferably) or departmental regulations to provide clear guidelines for forensic clinicians and administrators in their work. In that regard, the Virginia statute enacted at the conclusion of the pilot project[10] (see appendix E) may serve as a model in its detail and the underlying concern with defendants' rights. A second useful model, limited to competency to stand trial and in narrative rather than statutory form, has been provided by Roesch and Golding (1980, chap. 7).

In all of these considerations is the need to balance competing interests.

8. *See, e.g.,* Estelle v. Smith, 451 U.S. 454 (1981); Gibson v. Zahradnick, 581 F.2d 75 (4th Cir. 1978); United States v. Alvarez, 510 F.2d 1036 (3d Cir. 1975); United States *ex rel.* Edney v. Smith, 425 F. Supp. 1038 (E.D.N.Y. 1976).

9. Jackson v. Indiana, 406 U.S. 715 (1972), requires that defendants committed for restoration of competency "cannot be held more than a reasonable period of time necessary to determine whether there is a substantial probability that he will attain that capacity in the foreseeable future." *Id.* at 737-38.

10. Va. Code §§ 19.2-168.1 and 19.2-169.1 through 19.2-169.7 (Cum. Supp. 1982).

118

Conflicts between the defendant's and prosecution's interests in the gathering of incriminating evidence are obvious. Other conflicts are more subtle and perhaps more difficult from a policy perspective. For example, the defendant's right to evaluation and treatment (where the latter is relevant) in the least restrictive alternative may sometimes appear to be in conflict with the state's duty to take reasonable care in guarding the safety of other patients.[11] These dilemmas starkly pose the usefulness of careful consideration of the ethics and law of forensic evaluation. Particularly given the conflict of interests and roles that forensic clinicians themselves experience (see Melton et al., in press, chap. 3), representatives of the diverse interest groups (e.g., defense attorneys, prosecutors, patients' rights groups, and forensic clinicians themselves) should be asked in the policy formulation if those policies are in fact meeting their needs.[12]

PERSONNEL

Recommendation 5. A primary focus in the development of forensic services should be on intensive legally and psychologically sophisticated training in forensic issues. One of the clearest findings reported in this book is the existence of a specialty in forensic mental health (chapter 3). Trained forensic clinicians possess knowledge of relevant psychological research, clinical issues, and law that tends not to be shared by either general clinicians or legal authorities. A corollary to this conclusion is that training should be a major emphasis of forensic administrators, particularly given the obvious relationship between knowledge of the relevant legal standards and research literature and the quality of forensic evaluation. Although there has been an increase in programs designed to train new clinical psychologists with a forensic specialty (Grisso, Sales, & Bayless, 1982), such programs are still uncommon.[13] Therefore, it will be necessary to train mental health professionals, who already have general clinical competence, in the additional knowledge and skills to function as a forensic clinician.

11. *See* Restatement of Torts 2d §§ 319, 320.
12. It does not, of course, follow that a consensus must be reached before action can be taken. There are instances in which consensus is impossible or the apparently legally correct course is unpopular. However, the point here is that, at a minimum, the views of the parties concerned should be solicited and considered in decision making. As noted in the text, such feedback is also useful in ensuring that the system is working as intended.
13. As far as we are aware, predoctoral specialty training programs in forensic clinical psychology are available only at the University of Alabama, the University of Arizona, Hahnemann University/Villanova University School of Law, the University of Nebraska–Lincoln, Northwestern University, the University of Virginia, and the University of Wisconsin. It is possible to minor in forensic psychology at several other universities (e.g., California School of Professional Psychology, Berkeley; University of Illinois at Urbana-Champaign; Saint Louis University) (Melton, 1983b). Several of these programs are intended primarily to train clinical researchers rather than practitioners.

Recommendation 6. There should be continuing-education programs for fo-rensic clinicians, lawyers, and judges (see ABA, 1983, Std. 7-1.3 and com-mentary). Neither the law nor the state of knowledge is static, and dissemina-tion of changes in both is important in maintaining the quality of forensic services. If a clinician does an evaluation based on a legal standard that is no longer in force, the evaluation cannot be valid. Research suggests that changes in mental health law are unlikely to be transmitted quickly to mental health pro-fessionals most affected by them unless there is an active effort to disseminate the new law (see, e.g., Liss & Weinberger, 1983; Melton, 1981).

Similarly, lawyers and judges need to be kept informed about changes in the forensic evaluation system, research which is useful in making use of—or at-tacking—the opinion of mental health professionals, and relevant law. Just as special efforts must be made to ensure that forensic clinicians are kept abreast of the relevant law, dissemination of changes in the law is also not automatic for legal professionals (see, e.g., Wasby, 1976), especially those whose practice seldon includes cases involving criminal mental health law. This group probably includes most attorneys whose practice consists largely of criminal cases. Ac-tive efforts to disseminate new law are particularly important when the *system* of forensic evaluation is changed by the law in an area in which litigation is rare. For example, the restrictions that *Vitek v. Jones*[14] placed on procedures for transfer of prisoners to mental health facilities (Churgin, 1983)[15] have seldom been implemented (Monahan, Davis, Hartstone, & Steadman, 1983), at least in part because forensic administrators are often unaware of these constitutional requirements.[16] There is an inherent catch-22 in the dissemination and imple-mentation of law in that particular context. Lawyers seldom become involved in transfer of prisoners; hence, it is unlikely that the issue will be raised in a juris-diction where the *Vitek* procedures have not been implemented.[17]

The exact form of continuing education may vary. Virginia, for example, uses a widely distributed newsletter *Developments in Mental Health Law* which is published by the Institute of Law, Psychiatry and Public Policy at the University

14. 445 U.S. 480 (1980).

15. *Vitek* held that prisoners were entitled, at a minimum, to an administrative hearing before transfer to a mental health facility.

16. Our conclusion in this regard is based on anecdotal evidence. In conducting the content val-idation of our test of forensic knowledge (chapter 3), several members of the panel of experts ex-pressed surprise at a question on *Vitek*. They were apparently unaware of the case, and they indi-cated, as did the respondents in the survey by Monahan et al. (1983), that provisions were not in place in their states for hearings prior to transfer of prisoners to the mental health system.

17. We are aware that *Vitek* itself requires "qualified and independent assistance," rather than legally trained counsel. 445 U.S. at 500. However, the point here is that, without a procedural mecha-nism for challenging transfer of prisoners, there is no forum in which the issue is apt to be raised. Rather, the process of transfer is likely to remain hidden from public scrutiny (Hartstone, Steadman, & Monahan, 1982).

120

of Virginia with funds provided by the state Department of Mental Health and Mental Retardation. The institute sponsors an annual two-day symposium on mental health law, which attracts about two hundred mental health professionals and lawyers each year. The Institute also conducts periodic continuing-education workshops for particular groups (e.g., special justices who hear civil commitment cases), notably, semiannual workshops for clinicians trained and certified by the institute in forensic evaluation. Institute faculty make periodic visits to community mental health centers to talk with the forensic teams about problems they have encountered as well as new developments. Institute faculty also give lectures at continuing-education workshops of particular groups (e.g., trial judges).

There is, of course, an empirical question about the relative effectiveness of various formats for continuing education. Without such data, we offer no particular recommendation on formats that should be used; probably a combination of formats (as in the Virginia program) is optimal because the level of prior knowledge can vary with the particular audience.

Recommendation 7. Whether for basic training in forensic mental health or for continuing education, both lawyers and mental health professionals should be included as faculty. Forensic clinicians need to know the relevant legal standards and procedures, and lawyers' consultation or direct participation is essential in the development of forensic services. Forensic clinicians also need training in the techniques of, and research base for, forensic evaluation. Legal consumers of forensic services require an appreciation for both the relevant law and the prevailing state of the art. Also, both parties in this interdisciplinary interaction must have at least a basic understanding of the other discipline. Although we do not believe that the director of forensic services or forensic training must be a lawyer or a mental health professional (of whatever discipline), we do argue that it is important to have both lawyers and mental health professionals involved in training forensic clinicians.

Recommendation 8. Special incentives should be given for successful specialization in forensic mental health. Recruitment and retention of competent forensic clinicians have yet to be examined in detail. Forensic practice is probably viewed as undesirable by many clinicians (see Morse, 1982b, pp. 1053–1054), for reasons we have already acknowledged.[18] In view of the special skills and knowledge necessary for forensic practice (and the costs involved in

18. Professor Morse's conclusions are, as he admits, based on impressions rather than systematic evidence. However, there are several reasons to believe that forensic practice is near the bottom of the pecking order of mental health specialties. First, as noted in chapter 1, working conditions in forensic units have often been abysmal. Second, the double-agent status which forensic practice often

performing such training), financial incentives should be made available for performance of these duties. Also, recognition should be given in other ways (through job titles and "perks") of the expertise that competent forensic clinicians have attained.

Recommendation 9. The state should provide certification of expert forensic clinicians. The test for admissibility of experts' opinions concerns whether the specialized knowledge of the expert will assist the fact finder in decision making.[19] Like the assessments that forensic clinicians themselves make, the standard demands that judges take a *functional* approach to the question of whether the opinions of a particular expert or class of experts should be admitted into evidence. Accordingly, we have argued elsewhere (Melton et al., in press, chap. 1) that the range of mental health professionals permitted to testify as experts should be both broader and narrower than current practice allows in most jurisdictions (see also ABA, 1983, Stds. 7-3.10 and 7-3.11 and commentary). On the one hand, the operational definition of expert should be broader because neither the present studies nor previous research (see generally, Dix & Poythress, 1981) supports empirically a belief that medically trained or doctoral-level mental health professionals are more likely than clinicians with other educational backgrounds to be able to assist the fact finder in most cases. On the other hand, the range of mental health professionals permitted to testify should be narrower because the expert should possess the specialized knowledge (e.g., knowledge of the legal standard and relevant research concerning competency to stand trial) to be able to assist (and not mislead) the fact finder in the interpretation of the evidence.

The obvious practical difficulty with the approach that we are advocating is that it increases the complexity of the decision which the judge must make about the admissibility of a particular expert's opinion. Educational or professional credentials are easy to identify; evaluating the level of specialized knowledge that an expert possesses (and its probative or prejudicial value in the case) requires more extensive qualification of the expert and a more subjective and probably less reliable decision. Therefore, there are reasons of both efficiency and fairness to provide some objective measures of the expert's qualification on particular kinds of cases. Therefore, mental health professionals who successfully complete the state's forensic training and pass an examination on

---

creates (see Melton et al., in press, chap. 3) is uncomfortable for many mental health professionals. Third, forensic practice necessarily subjects one's work to public scrutiny in an adversary setting, a circumstance that some clinicians find stressful or even demeaning. Fourth, the clients of the forensic mental health system may themselves be perceived as undesirable. Fifth, forensic practice requires spending time away from "real" mental health work in the preparation for, and response to, legal proceedings.

19. Fed. R. Evid. 702.

the relevant body of specialized knowledge should be certified as forensic clinicians and presumed to qualify as experts on those types of cases extensively covered in the training program.

A side benefit of such an approach is that, consistent with recommendation 8, the title "certified forensic clinician" may come to carry a certain amount of prestige and serve as a recognition of the specialty. Thus, a certification process may be a low-cost way to recruit competent clinicians to forensic practice and provide an incentive for adequate investment of time and energy in the training program.

Although there are sound reasons for supporting a meaningful certification program, we do not support limiting qualification as experts to those who have been so certified. In some instances, mental health professionals may be able to provide assistance through their opinions about particular matters even though they have not received training in forensic evaluation. Consider, for example, a case in which a clinician has been treating a person for an extended period of time, and during the course of treatment, the person allegedly becomes involved in a crime. The treating clinician's opinions may provide especially probative evidence concerning the defendant's mental state near, if not at, the time of the offense. Also, some clinicians may have solid background in forensic mental health even though they have not completed a particular training program. Examples might be mental health professionals who are certified as diplomates by the American Board of Forensic Psychiatry or the American Board of Forensic Psychology or who have been trained in one of the few existing specialty programs. Provisions could, of course, be made for such clinicians to qualify for state certification by examination only (without taking the prescribed training) to ensure that they are familiar with standards and procedures prevailing in the particular jurisdiction.

To maximize incentives for community mental health centers to participate fully in the forensic service system, *referrals* for initial, publicly funded evaluations should be made only to certified forensic clinicians, even though, as noted above, a lack of such certification should not be a bar to qualification as an expert. To make use of other professional resources and to avoid alienation of professional groups, private clinicians might be permitted to enroll at their own expense in the training program to prepare for certification. Such a provision is especially desirable in communities in which there are few highly trained mental health professionals in the public sector.

MANAGEMENT

Recommendation 10. Provisions should be made for central coordination of forensic services. As Petrila (1981) has suggested, a major problem associated with community-based forensic services is that administration is necessarily more complex than in systems which rely primarily on a central forensic hospital. Simply put, there is more to administer when there is a range of programs and levels of services. Problems of coordination of services, development of standardized training, and control of quality are raised. Although these difficulties provide insufficient justification for failure to implement community-based services, it is important that they are recognized and that administrative structures are developed to deal with them. (Virginia did in fact find it necessary to create a position of director of forensic services in the Department of Mental Health and Mental Retardation.)

It is also important to provide interagency coordination. By definition, forensic services involve the mental health system in interaction with other agencies (e.g., sheriff's department, corrections department, court system).

In view of the need for coordination of forensic services, both internally and externally, there is a necessity for someone vested with that authority at the state level. Moreover, because of the nature of the specific tasks to be accomplished (e.g., establishment of interagency agreements, enforcement of standards for quality of services), it is desirable that the position be at the assistant-commissioner level so that the individual who possesses authority clearly has sufficient standing in the bureaucracy to be able to communicate easily with high-level administrators in other agencies. Also, because forensic services will cut across levels or types of mental health services (e.g., community services, hospitals), the director of forensic services needs to be at a level commensurate with, rather than subordinate to, the directors of these broad types of services, who will themselves typically be assistant commissioners. Finally, a high-level, independent position for forensic services in the mental health bureaucracy minimizes the possibility that funding for forensic services will be an afterthought in a division with other primary responsibilities.

Each forensic center should have a coordinator, too. Analogous to the job of the assistant commissioner, the local director of forensic services will have to ensure smooth working relationships with the various parties involved (e.g., prosecutor, clerk of court, judges, defense attorneys, probation staff). Representatives of the legal system need to know procedures for referral and whom to call in case of a problem. In appendix I, we have included materials circulated to such individuals by one community mental health center whose forensic program served several court jurisdictions. It provides a summary of the details with which local administrators must be concerned.

Recommendation 11. Ongoing attention should be given to management information services. As Steadman et al. (1982) discovered, many states are not even aware of the number of defendants who enter their forensic service programs or the auspices under which they enter. Without such information, it is impossible to do systematic program planning or evaluation. Well-developed data systems (see, e.g., Petrila & Hedlund, 1983) may also assist in identification of unanticipated problems (e.g., changes in referral patterns in a particular local jurisdiction) and determination of effects of changes in law or administrative policy. Such a need is present in human services generally, but it is especially acute in forensic services. The multiplicity of competing interests makes attempts to "sabotage" forensic service programs and unintended side effects especially common.

Of course, making the necessary management information accessible is not enough; it must also be analyzed. Program evaluation should be ongoing. In that regard, the substantial contribution that New York's Special Projects Office (directed by Henry Steadman) in the Office of Mental Health has made to understanding the interaction between the mental health and legal systems is exemplary of the utility of careful and continuing program evaluation.

FINANCING

Recommendation 12. Care should be taken to ensure the absence of economic disincentives for implementation of community-based services. As Kiesler (1982b) had convincingly shown, the national policy of provision of mental health services in the least restrictive alternative has yet to be translated into practice, largely because public funding mechanisms (e.g., Medicaid) still disproportionately reward use of inpatient services. Analogous disincentives can arise in forensic services. For example, as described in chapter 6, a major factor in the success of the Virginia program was the establishment of an interagency directive for the payment mechanism for outpatient forensic evaluations. Prior to the directive, local judges tended to refer evaluations to the forensic hospital rather than to local mental health professionals in part because the costs of the former were hidden. When local clinicians were engaged to perform evaluations, their fees were paid from the court's budget. The costs of hospitalization, on the other hand, were subsumed under the budget of the Department of Mental Health. Although inpatient evaluations were costly to the state, they were free to the referring agency, which therefore had a disincentive to use local clinicians.

Of course, circumvention of the system can also occur if fees are set too low. Apparently some community mental health clinics in Virginia perceived, for example, that screening evaluations were more profitable than comprehensive evaluations and consequently tended to refer cases to the forensic hospital for the latter. Similarly, clinics might be inclined to assign their least competent staff to forensic services if the income from the services is perceived as insufficient to justify use of highly trained staff.

Recommendation 13. Funding should be based on a mix of fees for services and lump-sum payments. It is difficult to be specific with respect to the mechanisms for funding because the fiscal structures available will vary across jurisdictions. For example, administrative relationships between state and local mental health agencies vary widely across states. We are reasonably confident, however, in suggesting a mix of fees for services and lump-sum contracts. Assuming that the fees are set at a level commensurate with the actual costs of performing the services, clinics will find it advantageous to perform services efficiently and quickly if they are reimbursed case by case. However, they are likely to find it disadvantageous economically to go beyond the provision of the report. Consequently, a lump-sum contract may be necessary to ensure that clinics do consultation and education, as well as direct delivery of services in individual cases (Dowell & Ciarlo, 1983). An initial lump-sum incentive may also be useful in covering the up-front costs of training and, therefore, enabling small clinics to put aside the necessary staff time prior to the receipt of significant fees for forensic services.

Summary

In our view, the case for community-based forensic services is compelling. They are substantially less costly, perhaps generally more effective, and certainly less restrictive than hospital-based services. Given the inherent intrusion of hospital-based services into constitutionally protected interests, the general finding that forensic services can be delivered at least as effectively in the community demands that states begin moving to community-based systems. There apparently is no state interest—certainly not a *compelling* one—justifying use of central, maximum-security facilities for forensic evaluations and, in many cases, forensic treatment. Moreover, establishment of a community-based forensic system is consistent with general trends in the mental health professions over the past two decades toward comprehensive community-based services.

At the same time, we recognize that establishment of community-based forensic services requires substantial planning and negotiation. Training programs must be instituted for the mental health professionals who will provide the services; the various interest groups involved must be courted and persuaded; and administrative and fiscal structures must be established. Careful attention must also be given to following and, as necessary, changing the legal standards and procedures governing forensic services. In short, although worthwhile, the development of high-quality, relatively unrestrictive forensic services is not a simple matter. Although this volume is not intended to be a handbook for implementing such services, we hope that it contributes to an understanding of the possibilities for interaction between courts and community mental health clinics. At a minimum, it provides some guideposts to the development of legally and psychologically sensible policies and procedures for forensic services.

Mental State at the Time of the Offense Screening Evaluation Format

I. Historical Information (from interview with defendant and available records)

A. Does the defendant have a history of prolonged bizarre behavior [i.e., delusions, hallucinations, looseness of association of ideas (thought processes incoherent and illogical), disturbance of affect (behavior disorganized, aggressive, intensely negativistic or withdrawn)]? If not, exclude:

   1. Organic brain syndromes of a progressive or chronic nature
     a. Dementia
     b. Organic personality syndrome

   2. Psychoses
     a. Schizophrenias
     b. Paranoid disorders
     c. Schizophreniform disorders
     d. Affective disorders

B. Does the defendant have a history of convulsive disorder (e.g., "fits" or "seizures")? If not, exclude most forms of epilepsy.

C. Has the defendant ever experienced a brief period of *uncharacteristic* bizarre behavior (i.e., delusions, hallucinations, sudden alterations in consciousness or motor functioning, sudden aggressive affectual discharge), not associated with psychoactive substance use? If not, exclude:

   1. Brief reactive psychosis

   2. Intermittent or isolated explosive disorder

   3. Automatism
     a. Post-concussion syndrome
     b. Temporal lobe (psychomotor) epilepsy
     c. Cerebral anoxia

128

4. Dissociative disorders
   a. Psychogenic fugue
   b. Sleepwalking

D. Does the defendant have a history of *episodic,* uncharacteristic bizarre behavior [i.e., delusions, hallucinations, looseness of association of ideas (thought processes incoherent and illogical), disturbance of affect (behavior disorganized, aggressive, intensely negativistic or withdrawn)], associated with psychoactive substance use? If not, exclude:

1. Withdrawal

2. Delirium or delusional disorder

3. Hallucinosis

E. Does the defendant exhibit signs of moderate or severe retardation? If not, exclude retardation.

If all of the above disorders are excluded, there is probably no evidence of "significant mental abnormality" approaching legal relevance, but further, more detailed evaluation regarding the degree of functional impairment at the time of the offense should always be performed. If one or more of the above disorders does or did exist, it is still necessary to determine whether it played a role in *significantly* impairing cognitive or volitional functioning at the time of the offense.

II. Offense Information

A. From the Defendant

1. Defendant's present "general" response to offense
   a. Cognitive perception of offense
   b. Emotional response

2. Detailed account of offense
   a. Evidence of intrapsychic stressors
      1. delusions
      2. hallucinations
   b. Evidence of external stressors
      1. provoking events
      2. fear or panic stimulants

     c. Evidence of altered state of consciousness
       1. alcohol-induced
       2. drug-induced
     d. Claimed amnesia
       1. partial
       2. complete

  3. Events leading up to offense
     a. Evidence of major changes in environment
       1. change in job status
       2. change in family status
     b. Relationship with victim
     c. Preparation for offense

  4. Post-offense response
     a. Behavior following act
     b. Emotional response to act
     c. Attempts to explain or justify act

B. From extrinsic sources

  1. Indictment, information or complaint

  2. Confessions, preliminary hearing transcripts, statements to the police

  3. Attorney's notes

  4. Autopsy reports (if relevant)

  5. Witness accounts

Though the above information will probably be sufficient to ascertain the existence of significant mental abnormality at the time of the offense, you should also assess *present* mental status to give you a fuller picture of the defendant's general psychological functioning. Of course, this may be accomplished in the course of earlier segments of the interview.

(Here a standard outline of a mental status examination is provided.)

House Joint Resolution No. 22

Requesting the Commissioner of Mental Health and Mental Retardation to establish a Forensic Evaluation Training and Research Center.

Agreed to by the House of Delegates, March 8, 1980
Agreed to by the Senate, March 8, 1980

WHEREAS, data provided by the Department of Mental Health and Mental Retardation demonstrates that a substantial proportion of criminal defendants committed to the Forensic Units of the State Hospitals for forensic evaluation do not require inpatient evaluation and do not need hospitalization; and

WHEREAS, the provisions of § 19.2-169 of the Code of Virginia now permit, but do not require, the courts to order the performance of forensic evaluations at appropriate community facilities; and

WHEREAS, the experiences of other states demonstrate that forensic evaluations of criminal defendants can be efficiently and competently performed by appropriately trained clinical personnel in community mental health clinics on an outpatient basis at less expense than in inpatient setting; and

WHEREAS, the personnel of the community mental health clinics have not been adequately trained to perform forensic evaluations; now, therefore, be it

RESOLVED by the House of Delegates, the Senate concurring, That the Commissioner of Mental Health and Mental Retardation (hereinafter referred to as the Commissioner) is requested to establish or contract for the establishment of a Forensic Evaluation Training and Research Center (hereinafter referred to as the Training and Research Center) for the following purposes:

1. To develop a plan for training community mental health professionals to perform forensic evaluations and to certify their qualifications and competency to do so;

2. To provide forensic training services for teams of community mental health professionals in jurisdictions selected by the Commissioner;

3. To develop clinical protocols and procedures for use by appropriately trained community mental health professionals to enable them (i) to efficiently screen and assess the competency of criminal defendants to stand trial, and (ii) to provide other appropriate psychological evaluations for the court; and

4. To compile the necessary information for evaluating the success of this program; and, be it

RESOLVED FURTHER, That the Commissioner shall make appropriate arrangements with selected community services boards:

1. To establish demonstration service projects in forensic evaluation; and

2. To work with the Training and Research Center to implement the objectives specified in the preceding paragraph.

These demonstration service projects shall:

1. include participation by designated mental health professionals in the training program developed by the Training and Research Center;

2. be coordinated with the courts to develop the necessary procedures for referring appropriate defendants for forensic evaluation;

3. conduct competency-to-stand trial evaluations for the courts as requested and without fee; and

4. conduct other forensic evaluations under conditions arranged with the Department of Mental Health and Mental Retardation and the courts; and, be it

RESOLVED FINALLY, That on or before September thirty, nineteen hundred eighty-two, the Commissioner shall prepare a report for the General Assembly describing the impact of this program. The report shall include a plan for providing community-based forensic evaluation and consultation services on a State-wide basis, as well as any necessary proposals for the revision of § 19.2-169 and other relevant sections of the Code of Virginia.

Model Format for Competency to Stand Trial Report[1]

NAME:

DOB:

DATE INTERVIEWED:

SUBJECT: COMPETENCY TO STAND TRIAL

SOURCES OF DATA (list):

(1) Interview(s)
(2) Documents
(3) Other sources

REFERRAL INFORMATION:

(1) Referral source
(2) Description of charge(s)
(3) Reason for referral (e.g., triggering behavior)

BACKGROUND INFORMATION:

(1) Prior psychiatric history
(2) Other relevant data from extrinsic sources

MENTAL STATUS EXAMINATION

Standard mental status exam, with special attention to the following, which have special significance for competency to stand trial:

(1) Degree of general orientation
(2) Capacity to form relationships
(3) Level of abstract thinking ability and memory
(4) Odd behavior
(5) Reaction to stress
(6) Suggestibility

1. Developed by Institute of Law, Psychiatry and Public Policy, University of Virginia.

UNDERSTANDING OF LEGAL SITUATION AND CAPACITY TO ASSIST IN OWN DEFENSE:

(1) Understanding of roles of courtroom personnel
(2) Understanding of courtroom procedures
(3) Comprehension of charges
(4) Understanding of alternative pleas
(5) Capacity to relate to attorney and participate in courtroom process
(6) Appropriate courtroom demeanor

CONCLUSIONS CONCERNING COMPETENCY TO STAND TRIAL:

(1) State: "It is our opinion that the defendant has the capacity to understand the proceedings against him and assist in his defense."
(2) If opinion is that the defendant is basically competent but that he needs education, indicate in which areas.
(3) If defendant likely to be found incompetent, address restorability issue (is he restorable, inpatient v. outpatient, etc.).

Report Rating Forms

Appendix D-1: Rating Sheet, Competency to Stand Trial

Report # _____

Rater Name _____

Please circle the number on each rating scale (from 1 to 9) which best reflects your assessment of the quality of the report according to each question (A through G).

A. How understandable is this report in terms of clear language versus mental health jargon?

Unclear, too much   Report clear, easily
jargon   understood
                        1 2 3 4 5 6 7 8 9

B. How familiar does the clinician appear to be with the appropriate legal criteria and issues?

Clinician unfamiliar,   Clinician familiar, used
used inappropriate   appropriate criteria
criteria
                        1 2 3 4 5 6 7 8 9

C. How clearly does the report characterize the defendant's capacity to understand the proceedings against him (her)?

Defendant's   Defendant's
understanding of the   understanding of the
proceedings not   proceedings described
described clearly   clearly
                        1 2 3 4 5 6 7 8 9

D. How clearly does the report characterize the defendant's capacity to assist in his (her) own defense?

Defendant's capacity to assist in own defense not described clearly

Defendant's capacity to assist in own defense described clearly

1 2 3 4 5 6 7 8 9

E. How adequately does the report explain the factual basis of the clinician's conclusions about the defendant's capacity to understand the proceedings and assist in own defense?

Factual basis not presented or unclear

Ample facts presented clearly

1 2 3 4 5 6 7 8 9

F. To what extent does this report provide the necessary information to assist the court in making a decision regarding the defendant's competency to stand trial?

Insufficient and/or inappropriate information provided

Sufficient and appropriate information provided

1 2 3 4 5 6 7 8 9

G. Please rate your impression of the overall quality of the report.

Poor report

Excellent report

1 2 3 4 5 6 7 8 9

H. We are interested in any additional comments you may have about the content, quality and style of the report. Please use the remainder of this page to make such comments.

Appendix D-2: Rating Sheet, Mental State at the Time of the Offense

Report # _____

Rater Name _____

Please circle the number on each rating scale (from 1 to 9) which best reflects your assessment of the quality of the report according to each question (A through G).

A. How understandable is this report in terms of clear language versus mental health jargon?

Unclear, too much
jargon

Report clear, easily
understood

1 2 3 4 5 6 7 8 9

B. How familiar does the clinician appear to be with the appropriate legal criteria and issues?

Clinician unfamiliar,
used inappropriate
criteria

Clinician familiar, used
appropriate criteria

1 2 3 4 5 6 7 8 9

C. How clearly does the report characterize the defendant's mental condition *at the time of the clinical interview?*

Mental condition not
described clearly

Mental condition
described clearly

1 2 3 4 5 6 7 8 9

D. How clearly does the report characterize the defendant's probable mental condition *at the time of the alleged crime?*

Mental condition not
described clearly

Mental condition
described clearly

1 2 3 4 5 6 7 8 9

E. How adequately does the report explain the factual basis for conclusions about mental state at the time of the alleged offense?

Factual basis not
presented or unclear

Ample facts presented
clearly

1 2 3 4 5 6 7 8 9

F. To what extent does this report provide the necessary information to assist the court in drawing conclusions about the defendant's criminal responsibility?

Insufficient and/or
inappropriate
information provided

Sufficient and
appropriate information
provided

1 2 3 4 5 6 7 8 9

G. Please rate your impression of the overall quality of this report.

Poor report   Excellent report

                 1 2 3 4 5 6 7 8 9

H. We are interested in any additional comments you may have about the content, quality and style of the report. Please use the remainder of this page to make such comments.

Appendix D-3: Rating Sheet, Sentencing Evaluation

Report #_____

Rater Name_____

Please circle the number on each rating scale (from 1 to 9) which best reflects your assessment of the quality of the report according to each question (A through H).

A. How understandable is this report in terms of clear language versus mental health jargon?

Unclear, too much   Report clear, easily
jargon   understood

                 1 2 3 4 5 6 7 8 9

B. Does the report respond appropriately to the referral questions?

Report does not focus   Report focuses
adequately on referral   adequately on referral
questions   questions

                 1 2 3 4 5 6 7 8 9

C. How clearly does the report characterize the defendant's mental condition *at the time of the clinical interview?*

Mental condition not   Mental condition
described clearly   described clearly

                 1 2 3 4 5 6 7 8 9

D. How adequately does the report describe psychological factors which may have been related to the defendant's behavior *at the time of the offense?*

Psychological factors not described adequately								Psychological factors described adequately

1 2 3 4 5 6 7 8 9

E. How adequately does the report explain the factual basis for clinical impressions of the relationship between psychological factors and the defendant's behavior at the time of the offense?

Factual basis not presented or unclear   Ample facts presented clearly

1 2 3 4 5 6 7 8 9

F. If requested by the referral source, does the report adequately present reasonable dispositional recommendations?

Dispositional recommendations not presented adequately   Dispositional recommendations presented adequately

1 2 3 4 5 6 7 8 9

G. To what extent does this report provide the psychological information necessary to assist the court in a sentencing determination?

Insufficient and/or inappropriate information provided   Sufficient and appropriate information provided

1 2 3 4 5 6 7 8 9

H. Please rate your impression of the overall quality of this report.

Poor report   Excellent report

1 2 3 4 5 6 7 8 9

I. We are interested in any additional comments you may have about the content, quality and style of the report. Please use the remainder of this page to make such comments.

Virginia Forensic Evaluation Law

Approved April 21, 1982

Be it enacted by the General Assembly of Virginia:

1. That §§ 19.2-175 and 19.2-176 of the Code of Virginia are amended and reenacted and that the Code of Virginia is amended by adding sections numbered 19.2-168.1 and 19.2-169.1 through 19.2-169.7 as follows:

§ 19.2-168.1. Evaluation on motion of the Commonwealth after notice.—A. If the attorney for the defendant gives notice pursuant to §19.2-168, and the Commonwealth thereafter seeks an evaluation of the defendant's mental state at the time of the offense, the court shall order such evaluation to be performed by one or more mental health professionals, one of whom is either a psychiatrist or a clinical psychologist with a doctorate degree. Evaluators who perform the evaluation shall report their opinion to the Commonwealth and the defense.

B. If the court finds, after hearing evidence presented by the parties, that the defendant has refused to cooperate with an evaluation requested by the Commonwealth, it may bar the defendant from presenting expert psychiatric or psychological evidence at trial on the issue of his mental state at the time of the offense.

§ 19.2-169.1. Raising question of competency to stand trial or plead; evaluation and determination of competency.—A. Raising competency issue; appointment of evaluators.—If, at any time after the attorney for the defendant has been retained or appointed and before the end of the trial, the court finds, upon hearing evidence or representations of counsel, that there is probable cause to believe that the defendant lacks substantial capacity to understand the proceedings against him or to assist his attorney in his own defense, the court shall order that a competency evaluation be performed by at least one psychiatrist or clinical psychologist who is qualified by training and experience to perform such evaluations.

B. Location of evaluation.—The evaluation shall be performed on an outpatient basis at a mental health facility or in jail unless the court specifically finds that outpatient evaluation services are unavailable or unless the results of out-

140

patient evaluation indicate that hospitalization of the defendant for evaluation on competency is necessary. If either finding is made, the court, under authority of this subsection, may order the defendant sent to a hospital designated by the Commissioner of Mental Health and Mental Retardation as appropriate for evaluations of persons under criminal charge. The defendant shall be hospitalized for such time as the director of the hospital deems necessary to perform an adequate evaluation of the defendant's competency, but not to exceed thirty days from the date of admission to the hospital.

C. Provision of information to evaluators.—The court shall require the attorney for the Commonwealth to provide to the evaluators appointed under subsection A any information relevant to the evaluation, including, but not limited to (i) a copy of the warrant or indictment; (ii) the names and addresses of the attorney for the Commonwealth, the attorney for the defendant, and the judge ordering the evaluation; (iii) information about the alleged crime; and (iv) a summary of the reasons for the evaluation request. The court shall require the attorney for the defendant to provide any available psychiatric records and other information that is deemed relevant.

D. The competency report.—Upon completion of the evaluation, the evaluators shall promptly submit a report in writing to the court and the attorneys of record concerning (i) the defendant's capacity to understand the proceedings against him; (ii) his ability to assist his attorney; and (iii) his need for treatment in the event he is found incompetent. No statements of the defendant relating to the time period of the alleged offense shall be included in the report.

E. The competency determination.—After receiving the report described in subsection D, the court shall promptly determine whether the defendant is competent to stand trial. A hearing on the defendant's competency is not required unless one is requested by the attorney for the Commonwealth ot the attorney for the defendant, or unless the court has reasonable cause to believe the defendant will be hospitalized under § 19.2-169.2. If a hearing is held, the party alleging that the defendant is incompetent shall bear the burden of proving by a preponderance of the evidence the defendant's incompetency. The defendant shall have the right to notice of the hearing, the right to counsel at the hearing and the right to personally participate in and introduce evidence at the hearing.

The fact that the defendant claims to be unable to remember the time period surrounding the alleged offense shall not, by itself, bar a finding of competency if the defendant otherwise understands the charges against him and can assist in his defense. Nor shall the fact that the defendant is under the influence of medication bar a finding of competency if the defendant is able to understand the charges against him and assist in his defense while medicated.

§ 19.2-169.2. Disposition when defendant found incompetent.—A. Upon finding pursuant to § 19.2-169.1 E that the defendant is incompetent, the court shall order that the defendant receive treatment to restore his competency on an outpatient basis or, if the court specifically finds that the defendant requires inpatient hospital treatment, at a hospital designated by the Commissioner of Mental Health and Mental Retardation as appropriate for treatment of persons under criminal charge. Any reports submitted pursuant to § 19.2-169.1 D shall be made available to the director of the treating facility.

B. If, at any time after the defendant is ordered to undergo treatment under paragraph A of this section, the director of the treatment facility believes the defendant's competency is restored, the director shall immediately send a report to the court as prescribed in § 19.2-169.1 D. The court shall make a ruling on the defendant's competency according to the procedures specified in § 19.2-169.1 E.

§ 19.2-169.3. Disposition of the unrestorable incompetent defendant.—A. If, at any time after the defendant is ordered to undergo treatment pursuant to § 19.2-169.2 A, the director of the treating facility concludes that the defendant is likely to remain incompetent for the foreseeable future, he shall send a report to the court so stating. The report shall also indicate whether, in the director's opinion, the defendant should be released, committed pursuant to § 37.1-67.3 of the Code, or certified pursuant to § 37.1-65.1 of the Code in the event he is found to be unrestorably incompetent. Upon receipt of the report, the court shall make a competency determination according to the procedures specified in § 19.2-169.1 E. If the court finds that the defendant is incompetent and is likely to remain so for the foreseeable future, it shall order that he be (i) released, (ii) committed pursuant to § 37.1-67.3, or (iii) certified pursuant to § 37-65.1. If the court finds the defendant incompetent but restorable to competency in the foreseeable future, it may order treatment continued until six months have elapsed from the date of the defendant's initial admission under § 19.2-169.2 A.

B. At the end of six months from the date of the defendant's initial admission under § 19.2-169.2 A if the defendant remains incompetent in the opinion of the director, the director shall so notify the court and make recommendations concerning disposition of the defendant as described above. The court shall hold a hearing according to the procedures specified in § 19.2-169.1 E and, if it finds the defendant unrestorably incompetent, shall order one of the dispositions described above. If the court finds the defendant incompetent but restorable to competency, it may order continued treatment under § 19.2-169.2 A for additional six-month periods, provided a hearing pursuant to § 19.2-169.1 E is held at the completion of each such period and the defendant continues to be incompetent but restorable to competency in the foreseeable future.

C. If not dismissed at an earlier time, charges against an unrestorable incompetent defendant shall be dismissed without prejudice on the date upon which his sentence would have expired had he been convicted and received the maximum sentence for the crime charged, or on the date five years from the date of his arrest for such charges, whichever is sooner.

§ 19.2-169.4. Litigating certain issues when the defendant is incompetent.— A finding of incompetency does not preclude the adjudication, at any time before trial, of a motion objecting to the sufficiency of the indictment, nor does it preclude the adjudication of similar legal objections which, in the court's opinion, may be undertaken without the personal participation of the defendant.

§ 19.2-169.5. Evaluation of sanity at the time of the offense; disclosure of evaluation results.—A. Raising issue of sanity at the time of offense; appointment of evaluators.—If, at any time after the attorney for the defendant has been retained or appointed and before trial, the court finds, upon hearing evidence or representations of counsel, that there is probable cause to believe that the defendant's actions during the time of the alleged offense may have been affected by mental disease or defect, the court shall order that an evaluation of the defendant's sanity at the time of the offense be performed by at least one psychiatrist or psychologist with a doctorate degree in clinical psychology who is qualified by training and experience to perform such evaluations.

B. Location of evaluation.—The evaluation shall be performed on an outpatient basis, at a mental health facility or in jail, unless the court specifically finds that outpatient services are unavailable, or unless the results of the outpatient evaluation indicate that hospitalization of the defendant for further evaluation of his mental state at the time of the offense is necessary. If either finding is made, the court, under authority of this subsection, may order that the defendant be sent to a hospital designated by the Commissioner as appropriate for evaluation of the defendant under criminal charge. The defendant shall be hospitalized for such time as the director of the hospital deems necessary to perform an adequate evaluation of the defendant's mental state at the time of the offense, but not to exceed thirty days from the date of admission to the hospital.

C. Provision of information to evaluators.—The court shall require the party making the motion for the evaluation, and such other parties as the court deems appropriate, to provide to the evaluators appointed under subsection A any information relevant to the evaluation, including, but not limited to (i) copy of the warrant or indictment, (ii) the names and addresses of the attorney for the Commonwealth, the attorney for the defendant and the judge ordering the evaluation, (iii) information pertaining to the alleged crime, including statements by the defendant made to the police and transcripts of preliminary hearings, if any, (iv) a summary of the reasons for the evaluation request, and (v) any available psychiatric, psychological, medical or social records that are deemed relevant.

D. The report.—The evaluators shall prepare a full report concerning the defendant's mental state at the time of the offense, including whether he may have had a significant mental disease or defect which rendered him insane at the time of the offense. The evaluators shall also prepare a summary of their conclusions which shall not include any statements by the defendant about the time period of the alleged offense. The full report and the summary shall be prepared within the time period designated by the court, said period to include the time necessary to obtain and evaluate the information specified in subsection C.

E. Disclosure of evaluation results.—The summary of the evaluators' conclusions described in subsection D shall be sent to the attorney for the Commonwealth and the court. The full report described in subsection D shall be sent solely to the attorney for the defendant and shall be deemed to be protected by the lawyer-client privilege; however, the Commonwealth shall be given the report and the results of any other evaluation of the defendant's mental state at the time of the offense after the attorney for the defendant gives notice of an intent to present psychiatric or psychological evidence pursuant to § 19.2-168 of the Code.

§ 19.2-169.6. Emergency treatment prior to trial.—A. Any defendant who is not subject to the provisions of § 19.2-169.2 may be hospitalized for psychiatric treatment prior to trial if the circuit or general district court judge with jurisdiction over the defendant's case, or a judge designated by such judge, finds clear and convincing evidence that the defendant: (i) is being properly detained in jail prior to trial; (ii) is mentally ill and imminently dangerous to self or others in the opinion of a qualified mental health professional; and (iii) requires treatment in a hospital rather than the jail in the opinion of a qualified mental health professional. The attorney for the defendant shall be notified that the court is considering hospitalizing the defendant for psychiatric treatment and shall have the opportunity to challenge the findings of the qualified mental health professional. If the court decides to hospitalize the defendant, it shall also indicate in its order whether the admitting hospital should evaluate the defendant's competency to stand trial and his mental state at the time of the offense pursuant to §§ 19.2-169.1 and 19.2-169.5.

B. A defendant subject to this section shall be treated at a hospital designated by the Commissioner as appropriate for treatment and evaluation of persons under criminal charge. The director of the hospital, within thirty days of the defendant's admission, shall send a report to the court with jurisdiction over the defendant addressing the defendant's continued need for treatment as mentally ill and imminently dangerous to self or others and, if so ordered by the court, the defendant's competency to stand trial, pursuant to § 19.2-169.1 D, and his men-

144

tal state at the time of the offense, pursuant to § 19.2-169.5 D. Based on this report, the court shall either (i) find the defendant incompetent to stand trial pursuant to § 19.2-169.1 E and proceed accordingly, (ii) order that the defendant be discharged from custody pending trial, (iii) order that the defendant be returned to jail pending trial, or (iv) make other appropriate disposition, including dismissal of charges and release of the defendant.

C. A defendant may not be hospitalized longer than thirty days under this section unless the court which has criminal jurisdiction over him, or a court designated by such court, holds a hearing at which the defendant shall be represented by an attorney and finds clear and convincing evidence that the defendant continues to be (i) mentally ill, (ii) imminently dangerous to self or others, and (iii) in need of psychiatric treatment in a hospital. Hospitalization may be extended in this manner for periods of sixty days, but in no event may such hospitalization be continued beyond trial, nor shall such hospitalization act to delay trial, so long as the defendant remains competent to stand trial.

§ 19.2-169.7. Disclosure by defendant during evaluation or treatment; use at guilt phase of trial.—No statement or disclosure by the defendant concerning the alleged offense made during a competency evaluation ordered pursuant to § 19.2-169.1, a mental state at the time of the offense evaluation ordered pursuant to § 19.2-169.5, or treatment ordered pursuant to § 19.2-169.2 or § 19.2-169.6 may be used against the defendant at trial as evidence or as a basis for such evidence, except on the issue of his mental condition at the time of the offense after he raises the issue pursuant to § 19.2-168.

§ 19.2-175. Expenses of physicians, etc.—Each expert or physician or clinical psychologist skilled in the diagnosis of insanity or mental retardation or other physician appointed by the court to render professional service pursuant to §§ 19.2-168.1, 19.2-169.1, 19.2-169.5 or paragraphs (1) and (2) of § 19.2-181, who is not regularly employed by the Commonwealth of Virginia except by the University of Virginia School of Medicine and the Medical College of Virginia, shall receive a reasonable fee for each such examination and report thereof to the court. The fee shall be determined in each instance by the court which made the appointment in accordance with the relevant regulations promulgated by the Department of Mental Health and Mental Retardation. In no event shall a fee exceed $200, but in addition if any such expert be required to appear as a witness in any hearing held pursuant to such sections, he shall receive mileage and a fee of fifty dollars for each day during which he is required so to serve. Itemized account of expense, duly sworn to, must be presented to the court, and when allowed shall be certified to the Supreme Court for payment out of the state treasury, and be charged against the appropriation made to pay criminal charges. Allowance for the fee and for the per ciem authorized shall also be made by order of the court, duly certified to the Supreme Court for payment out of the appropriation to pay criminal charges.

§ 19.2-176. Determination of insanity after conviction but before sentence.— If, after conviction and before sentence of any person, the judge presiding at the trial shall find reasonable ground to question such person's mental state, he may order an evaluation of such person's mental state by at least one psychiatrist or clinical psychologist who is qualified by training and experience to perform such evaluations. If the judge, based on the evaluation, and after hearing representations of the defendant's counsel, finds clear and convincing evidence that the defendant (i) is mentally ill, and (ii) requires treatment in a mental hospital rather than the jail, he may order the defendant hospitalized in a facility designated by the Commissioner as appropriate for treatment of persons convicted of crime. The time such person is confined to such hospital shall be deducted from any term for which he may be sentenced to any penal institution, reformatory or elsewhere.

2. That §§ 19.2-169, 19.2-170, 19.2-171, 19.2-172, 19.2-173, 19.2-174 and 19.2-182.1 of the Code of Virginia are repealed. □

Interagency Agreement concerning the Pilot Project

November 21, 1980

Memorandum

To:
General District Court Judges
Circuit Court Judges
Probation Officers
City and County Sheriffs of the Commonwealth
Directors, Community Mental Health Centers

From:
Office of the Executive Secretary of the Supreme Court
Office of the Attorney General
Department of Mental Health and Mental Retardation

Subject:
Outpatient Forensic Evaluations for Adult[1] Criminal Courts

INTRODUCTION

On January 16, 1980, the General Assembly passed House Joint Resolution 22, directing the Commissioner of Mental Health and Mental Retardation to establish a Forensic Evaluation Training and Research Center. The Assembly had found that (1) a substantial proportion of criminal defendants committed to Central and Southwestern State Hospitals did not require inpatient evaluation; (2) that other states had successfully established a system for conducting forensic evaluations on an outpatient basis, at less expense; and (3) that implementation of a similar program in the Commonwealth of Virginia required training of personnel at community mental health clinics. The Department has established the Center under the aegis of the Institute of Law, Psychiatry and Public Policy at the University of Virginia to devise a demonstration project

---

1. Procedures for ordering evaluations of juveniles charged with delinquency offenses will be the subject of a forthcoming directive.

which will provide forensic training to mental health professionals, implement a system for utilizing outpatient evaluations and monitor the success of the program.

FORENSIC TRAINING PROGRAM

In order to carry out its mandate, the Center has selected six target Community Mental Health Centers (CMHCs) to participate in a two-year demonstration project. These CMHCs are located in Alexandria, Charlottesville, Portsmouth, Radford, Richmond and Roanoke. Between October 15, 1980, and April 15, 1981, teams of psychiatrists, psychologists, social workers and other mental health professionals from these CMHCs will be trained to perform forensic evaluations for the courts in their catchment areas. Specifically, they will be trained to assess a defendant's competency to stand trial, to evaluate his/her mental state at the time of an alleged offense (MSO), and to assess an offender's amenability to treatment for rehabilitation.

The type of examination (and the fee for the CMHC's services) wil depend upon the court order in a particular case.[2] There will be three types of examinations.

1. *Routine Competency and MSO Screening and Examinations* will be all that is required in most cases. The CMHCs will determine whether the defendant is competent to stand trial and will recommend appropriate treatment if the defendant's mental condition warrants it; if the court specifically so orders, the CMHCs will also provide a general assessment of the defendant's mental state at the time of the alleged offense, determining whether the defendant exhibits any signs of significant mental abnormality and, if so, whether further evaluation is indicated.

2. *Comprehensive MSO Evaluations* will provide in-depth evaluation of the offender's psychological functioning at the time of the alleged offense.

3. *Pre-sentence Evaluations* will provide comprehensive assessment of the offender's mental/behavioral status and, where appropriate, will make specific therapeutic or rehabilitative recommendations. Given the limited amount of professional staff and time available, courts should endeavor to restrict their pre-sentence referrals to those cases in which clinical input is likely to be most useful.[3] Such cases might include:

2. Staff from the Forensic Evaluation Training and Research Center, in conjunction with the Attorney General's Office, will provide model orders which will be responsive to the differences between evaluations and between defense and prosecution originated requests.

3. When the probation office prepares a pre-sentence report under § 19.2-399, it would be helpful in this regard if it included in the report a recommendation to the court as to whether a psychological evaluation is warranted. If such a recommendation is made, and the court agrees, the report should be attached to the court order.

148

a. Capital offenses, which involve the special sentencing provisions of § 19.2-264.4;

b. Offenses involving "sexual abnormality" (e.g., rape, attempted rape, exhibitionism) which may trigger the provisions of § 19.2-300;

c. Offenses committed by an individual between 17 and 21, or who was a juvenile certified for trial as an adult, who meets the requirements of § 19.2-311 and is therefore eligible for "indeterminate commitment" to the Department of Corrections, under the conditions specified in §§ 19.2-311, 19.2-312, and 19.2-313.

COURT REFERRALS: TIMETABLE

When training is completed, the courts in the catchment areas of the six target CMHCs will begin referring adult defendants and juvenile defendants certified for trial as adults to the appropriate CMHCs, according to the following timetable:

1. Beginning January 12, 1981 for courts in the catchment areas of the Alexandria CMHC, Richmond CMHC and Roanoke Valley CMHC and beginning February 2, 1981 for courts in the catchment areas of the Region X MHC (Charlottesville), New River Valley (Radford), and Maryview Hospital CMHC (Portsmouth), *all* competency and MSO screening examinations ordered under § 19.2-169 shall be referred to the appropriate CMHC.

2. Beginning March 16, 1981 for courts in the catchment areas of Alexandria CMHC, Richmond CMHC and Roanoke Valley CMHC and beginning April 27, 1981 for courts in the catchment areas of Region X MHC (Charlottesville), New River Valley (Radford), and Maryview Hospital CMHC (Portsmouth), the CMHCs will be available to provide comprehensive MSO evaluations and presentence evaluations, though other evaluators may also be utilized for these types of examinations. Until the indicated dates, Central State Hospital will be available to provide comprehensive MSO evaluations.

If the evaluation is to be performed at the CMHC rather than the jail, the appropriate sheriff's office shall be responsible for transporting the defendant to the evaluation CMHC and providing the necessary security.

REIMBURSEMENT

Upon submission to the court of a written report based on its evaluation, the CMHC shall be entitled to reimbursement for each specifically ordered evaluation according to the following schedule:

1. Competency and MSO Screening Examination
(Considered to be one report) $100.00

2. Comprehensive MSO Evaluations	$200.00
3. "Pre-sentence" Evaluations:	$100.00

or, if there has been no prior
comprehensive MSO evaluation: $200.00

Reimbursement for competency and MSO screening evaluations and comprehensive MSO evaluations of indigent defendants (i.e., those with court-appointed attorneys) shall be made under § 19.2-175, which authorizes payments of up to $200.00 per evaluation for psychological evaluations.[4] Courts will make reimbursement for pre-sentence reports under § 19.2-332.

Defendants with retained attorneys will be required to pay for any evaluations that they request. In such cases, the CMHCs will be responsible for collecting from the defendant.

The above schedule does not apply to evaluations performed by evaluating entities other than designated CMHCs.

Reimbursement for testimony deriving from any evaluation shall be allocated separately under the provisions of § 19.2-175.

CONCLUSION

The Office of the Executive Secretary of the Supreme Court of Virginia, the Attorney General, and the Department of Mental Health and Mental Retardation support the implementation of H.J.R. 22 through the above described demonstration project. It is believed that this project will increase the quality of the forensic services provided to the courts, decrease the costs and delays occasioned by referral to distant state hospitals,[5] and make it possible for the state forensic units to concentrate on those individuals who truly require inpatient care. To realize these benefits, it is imperative that the judiciary and the mental health profession cooperate fully with each other. Enthusiastic support of all aspects of this demonstration project is essential.

In order to facilitate understanding of the project, staff from the Forensic

4. Section 19.2-175 provides that such payments shall not be paid to state employees. It is the opinion of the Attorney General's Office that mental health professionals employed by CMHCs are not state employees.

5. The average cost per patient at Central State Hospital is between $60.00 and $100.00 per day. The average stay there is 20 days. An estimated 700 patients are hospitalized per year under § 19.2-169. The cost of hospitalization under § 19.2-169 is thus well over $1 million per year. This figure does not include transportation costs incurred by the state police and communication costs incurred by the courts and attorneys. The total estimated cost of the program described in this directive is $300,000 per year. Moreover, it is felt that the time spent transporting the defendants to Central State and evaluating them there will be drastically reduced by a system utilizing local evaluations.

Evaluation Training and Research Center and the Attorney General's Office will contact individually each court involved by December 30, 1980.

ROBERT N. BALDWIN, Executive Secretary, Supreme Court

LEO E. KIRVEN, JR., M.D., Commissioner, Department of Mental Health and Mental Retardation

PAUL A. SINCLAIR, Assistant Attorney General

VA. CODE §§ 19.2-169.1, 19.2-169.5 File No. ....

ORDER FOR PSYCHOLOGICAL EVALUATION

COURT NAME AND ADDRESS

Commonwealth of Virginia V. ....

Type of Evaluation and Report

☐ COMPETENCY TO STAND TRIAL: It appearing to the Court, on motion of
   ☐ Commonwealth's Attorney ☐ defendant's attorney ☐ the Court
and upon hearing evidence or representations of counsel, that there is probable cause to believe that the defendant lacks substantial capacity to understand the proceedings against him or to assist in his own defense, the Court therefore appoints the evaluator(s) listed below to evaluate the defendant and to submit a report, on or before the date shown below, to this Court, the Commonwealth's Attorney, and the defendant's attorney, concerning: (1) the defendant's capacity to understand the proceedings against him; (2) his ability to assist his attorney; and (3) his need for treatment in the event that he is found to be incompetent. No statement of the defendant relating to the time period of the alleged offense shall be included in the report.

☐ MENTAL STATE AT THE TIME OF THE OFFENSE: It appearing to the Court, on motion of
   ☐ Commonwealth's Attorney ☐ defendant's attorney ☐ the Court
and upon hearing evidence or representations of counsel, that there is probable cause to believe that the defendant's actions during the time of the alleged offense may have been affected by mental disease or defect, the Court therefore appoints the evaluator(s) listed below to evaluate the defendant and submit a report, on or before the date shown below, to the defendant's attorney, and a summary of the report (which shall not include any statements by the defendant about the alleged offense) to the Court and the Commonwealth's Attorney, concerning the defendant's mental state at the time of the offense, including whether he may have had a significant mental disease or defect which rendered him insane at the time of the offense. If further evaluation on this issue is necessary, the evaluator(s) shall so state.

Designation of Evaluator(s)

It appearing to the Court that the evaluation
☐ can be conducted on an outpatient basis in jail or a mental health facility
☐ must be conducted on an inpatient basis because:
   ☐ no outpatient services are available
   ☐ the results of outpatient evaluation (copy attached) indicate that hospitalization for further evaluation is necessary
   ☐ a court of competent jurisdiction has found, pursuant to Va. Code §§ 19.2-169.6 or 37.1-67.3, that the defendant requires emergency treatment on an inpatient basis at this time
The Court therefore appoints the following evaluator(s) to conduct the evaluation:

☐ ....
OUTPATIENT EVALUATOR(S) (NAME(S) AND TITLE(S) OR NAME OF FACILITY
☐ qualified staff at a hospital to be designated by the Commissioner of Mental Health and Mental Retardation or his designee. Hospitalization for evaluation shall not extend beyond 30 days from the date of admission.

DUE DATE AND TIME: ....

The Court further orders that the Commonwealth's Attorney and the defendant's attorney to forward appropriate background information to the evaluator(s) as required by law.

TO EVALUATORS AND ATTORNEYS: See reverse for additional instructions.

....
DATE   JUDGE

FORM DC-342 3/82 (114:0-301 7/82)   File No. ....

ORDER FOR PSYCHOLOGICAL EVALUATION

Model Orders

ADDITIONAL INSTRUCTIONS TO EVALUATOR(S) AND ATTORNEYS

Providing Background Information

1. *Competency to Stand Trial: Prior to an evaluation of competency to stand trial, the Commonwealth's Attorney must forward to the evaluator(s):*

   (a) *a copy of the warrant*
   (b) *the names and addresses of the Commonwealth's Attorney, the defendant's attorney, and the judge ordering the evaluation*
   (c) *information about the alleged crime*
   (d) *a summary of the reasons for the evaluation request*

   The defendant's attorney must provide any available psychiatric records and other information that is deemed relevant. Va. Code § 19.2-169.1 (C).

2. *Mental State at the Time of the Offense: Prior to an evaluation of mental state at the time of the offense, the party making the motion for the evaluation must forward to the evaluator(s):*

   (a) *a copy of the warrant*
   (b) *the names and addresses of the Commonwealth's Attorney, the defendant's attorney, and the judge ordering the evaluation*
   (c) *information pertaining to the alleged crime, including statements by the defendant made to the police and transcripts of preliminary hearings, if any*
   (d) *a summary of the reasons for the evaluation request*
   (e) *any available psychiatric, psychological, medical or social records that are deemed relevant.*

   Va. Code § 19.2-169.5 (C).

Use of Information Obtained During Evaluation

   No statement of disclosure by the defendant concerning the alleged offense made during the evaluation may be used against the defendant at trial as evidence, or as a basis for such evidence, except on the issue of his/her mental condition at the time of the offense after the defendant raises the issue pursuant to § 19.2-168 of the Code of Virginia. Va. Code § 19.2-169.7.

DC-342 (REVERSE) 3 82

152

VA. CODE § 19.2-169.6 File No. . . . .

ORDER FOR EMERGENCY HOSPITAL TREATMENT
PENDING TRIAL

. . . .
COURT NAME AND ADDRESS

Commonwealth of Virginia vs. . . . .

It appearing to the Court, by clear and convincing evidence, which the defendant's attorney has had the opportunity to challenge, that the defendant is

(1) properly detained in jail prior to trial and is not presently eligible to be released on personal recognizance or on bond; and

(2) is mentally ill and imminently dangerous to
☐ self
☐ others
in the opinion of a qualified mental health professional, as indicated in the attached report; and

(3) requires treatment in a hospital rather than the jail in the opinion of a qualified mental health professional, as indicated in the attached report,

the Court therefore ORDERS that the defendant be committed for psychiatric treatment to a hospital to be designated by the Commissioner of Mental Health and Mental Retardation or his designee for a period not to exceed 30 days from the date of admission.

Within 30 days of the defendant's admission, the director of the hospital shall send a report to the Court addressing the defendant's continued need for treatment as mentally ill and imminently dangerous to self or others.

☐ See attached Order for Psychological Evaluation.

. . . .
DATE   JUDGE

FORM DC-340 3/82 (114:0-301 6/82)

File No. . . . .

ORDER FOR EMERGENCY HOSPITAL TREATMENT
PENDING TRIAL

VA. CODE §§19.2-169.2, 19.2-169.3   File No. ....

ORDER FOR TREATMENT OF INCOMPETENT DEFENDANT

....
COURT NAME AND ADDRESS

Commonwealth of Virginia vs. ....

The Court having found, pursuant to §19.2-169.1(E) of the Code of Virginia, that the Defendant is incompetent to stand trial, and having found further, based on the attached report or other evidence, that the defendant can be treated to restore his competency

☐ on an outpatient basis in jail or through a local mental health facility
☐ solely on an inpatient basis in a hospital

the Court therefore ORDERS

☐ ....
NAME OF OUTPATIENT THERAPIST OR FACILITY

☐ qualified staff at a hospital to be designated by the Commissioner of Mental Health and Mental Retardation or his designee

to treat the Defendant in an effort to restore him to competency.

If, at any time after treatment commences, the director of the treatment facility believes the Defendant's competency is restored, the director shall immediately send a report to the Court concerning (1) the Defendant's capacity to understand the proceedings against him and (2) his ability to assist his attorney.

If, at any time after treatment commences, the director of the treatment facility concludes that the defendant is likely to remain incompetent for the foreseeable future, he shall send a report to the court so stating and indicating whether, in the director's opinion, the Defendant (1) should be released from state custody; (2) committed pursuant to §37.1-67.3 of the Code of Virginia; or (3) certified pursuant to §37.1-65.1 of the Code of Virginia.

If the defendant has not been restored to competency by six months from the date of the commencement of treatment, the director of the treating facility shall send a report to the court so stating and indicating whether, in the director's opinion, the Defendant remains restorable to competency or whether the Defendant (1) should be released from state custody; (2) committed pursuant to § 37.1-67.3 of the Code of Virginia or (3) certified pursuant to § 37.1-65.1 of the Code of Virginia.

....
DATE   JUDGE

File No. ....

FORM DC-345 3/82 (114:0-301 6/82)

ORDER FOR TREATMENT OF INCOMPETENT DEFENDANT

Interagency Memorandum on Fees

To:
Circuit Court Judges
General District Court Judges
Commonwealth's Attorneys
City and County Sheriffs of the Commonwealth
Directors, Community Mental Health Centers

From:
Office of the Executive Secretary of the Supreme Court of Virginia
Office of the Attorney General of Virginia
Department of Mental Health and Mental Retardation

Subject:
Fee Schedule for Local Mental Evaluations of Criminal Defendants Ordered
Pursuant to § 19.2-169 of the Code of Virginia (as amended July 1, 1982).

INITIATION OF STATE-WIDE LOCAL OUTPATIENT EVALUATION SYSTEM

Over the past year, the Department of Mental Health and Mental Retardation,
through the Forensic Evaluation Training and Research Center at the University
of Virginia, has conducted studies to determine the feasibility of training community mental health professionals to perform evaluations for the courts. The
results of this research indicate that outpatient evaluations conducted by such
professionals result in reduced admissions to State hospitals, at a significant
savings to the State, *with no apparent decline in the quality of the evaluations.*
Given the positive findings of these studies, the Department has instructed the
Center to train mental health professionals from selected Community Mental
Health Centers (CMHCs) to perform evaluations of competency to stand trial
and mental state at the time of the offense. The eventual aim is to make outpatient evaluations available to each judicial circuit by March 1, 1984. This step
coincides with the passage of amendments to § 19.2-169 (Senate Bill No. 417)
which require the court to initially obtain such evaluations at the local level (if

they are available) instead of sending the defendant to the hospital for evaluation. (See §§ 19.2-169.1(B) and 19.2-169.5(B), *effective July 1, 1982.*)

Judges, lawyers, and sheriffs will be notified by the Center when mental health professionals from the CMHC servicing their area have been trained and are available to perform forensic evaluations. After such notification, when the court orders an evaluation of either competency to stand trial or mental state at the time of the offense, it shall, pursuant to §§ 19.2-169.1(B) and 19.2-169.5(B) of the Code of Virginia, utilize the CMHC rather than the hospital.[1] Although, in some cases, the community mental health professionals may indicate that a defendant needs further evaluation in a hospital setting, the experience in the experimental jurisdictions has been that most evaluations can be completed at the local level with significant savings in both hospital care and transportation costs.

These evaluations will be performed either at the jail or at the CMHC facility. If the latter, the appropriate sheriff's office is responsible for transporting the defendant to the evaluation and providing the necessary security.

REIMBURSEMENT FOR EVALUATIONS OF INDIGENT DEFENDANTS

Section 19.2-175 of the Code of Virginia[2] authorizes payment of up to $200.00 per mental evaluation and report, "in accordance with the relevant regulations promulgated by the Department of Mental Health and Mental Retardation."[3] This memorandum establishes the fee schedule for mental evaluations of indigent criminal defendants that are performed by CMHCs until such time as such regulations are promulgated by the Department.

Upon submission of a written evaluation report on an indigent defendant to the court or to the initiating party, the CMHC shall be entitled to reimbursement according to the following schedule:[4]

1. Competency evaluation $100.00

1. If the court is already using local services and is satisfied with them, it may, of course, continue to rely on these services. In these jurisdictions, the CMHC will merely provide another local resource for the court. Eventually, however, the Department hopes that the courts will rely on personnel affiliated with the CMHCs because they have been specifically trained to perform such evaluations and can develop a permanent relationship with the court.

2. Section 19.2-175 provides that such payments shall not be made to State employees. It is the opinion of the Attorney General's Office that mental health professionals employed by CMHCs are not State employees.

3. Effective July 1, 1982.

4. This schedule supercedes the schedule promulgated by the Department on November 20, 1980, for the six experimental jurisdictions.

2. Competency evaluation *plus* preliminary or "screening"
evaluation of mental state at the time of the offense $150.00

3. Comprehensive evaluation of mental state at the time of the
offense $200.00

4. Pre-sentence evaluation:
a. Only $200.00
b. If competency or mental state at the time of the offense
evaluation already performed $100.00

Reimbursement of evaluators not affiliated with a CMHC shall be governed by the provisions of § 19.2-175 and the court's customary fee schedule.

Questions about reimbursement should be directed to Robert N. Baldwin, Executive Secretary of the Supreme Court of Virginia. Questions concerning the availability and capabilities of the CMHCs should be directed to Donald K. Jones, M.D., Director, Medicolegal Services, Department of Mental Health and Mental Retardation, P.O. Box 1797, Richmond, Virginia 23214 or by phone at (804) 786-1332.

ROBERT N. BALDWIN, Executive Secretary
Supreme Court of Virginia

JOSEPH J. BEVILACQUA, Ph.D., Commissioner
Department of Mental Health and Mental
Retardation

MASTON T. JACKS, Deputy Attorney General

cc: Directors, State Mental Hospitals

Model Format for Referral Brochure[1]

FORENSIC EVALUATION SERVICES

Mental Health Services Center of Midtown Area

TO ARRANGE EVALUATION: Please call the Administrative Offices at 999-9999. We prefer several days' notice in order to adjust staff schedules to accommodate the evaluation.

LOCATION: The evaluations will preferably be conducted at the Midtown Office which is located at 100 First Street (map attached). The evaluation will be conducted in an interior office with no windows and only one exit to facilitate security arrangements. Persons in custody may wear leg chains. If necessary in certain cases a defendant may be evaluated while in the Central County Jail. It may also be possible for persons in custody in the other local jails to be evaluated in the jail facility.

TIME OF EVALUATION: The competency evaluation should be expected to take two or two and one-half hours to conduct. The presentence evaluation and evaluation of mental status at the time of the offense will vary in time required depending on the individual case and whether or not we have examined the defendant previously. We will attempt to give the court an estimate of length of time for each case.

REPORTS: Reports will be returned to the appropriate persons in the judicial system within two weeks of the evaluation.

TO BOARD persons in custody overnight, Central County Sheriff John Smith has graciously offered the facilities of the Central County Jail. If you desire to have the prisoner boarded overnight, the Central County Jail should be notified in

---

1. This is a modified version of the brochure provided to judges, attorneys, sheriffs, and clerks of court by the Mental Health Services of the New River Valley, Radford, Virginia. Acknowledgment is due the center's forensic team coordinator, Michael B. Brown.

advance by calling (888) 888-8888. The jail is located at 100 Main Street. They will give you directions over the phone.

IN CASE OF QUESTIONS OR CONCERNS, please call the Administrative Offices (999-9999) and ask for Dr. George Williams, Forensic Team Leader, or Dr. Jane Jones, Center Director.

CLINICAL STAFF: The Center staff who will be conducting these evaluations have received intensive training through the [name of forensic institute], in addition to their clinical training. Project Staff includes [here list all staff members, their degrees, internship training, position in the CMHC, etc.]

References

American Bar Association. (1983). *Tentative draft criminal justice mental health standards.* Washington, DC: Author.

American Psychiatric Association. (1982). *Statement on the insanity defense.* Washington, DC: Author.

American Psychological Association. (1981). Ethical principles of psychologists. *American Psychologist, 36,* 633–638.

Arenella, P. (1977). The diminished capacity and diminished responsibility defenses: Two children of a doomed marriage. *Columbia Law Review, 77,* 827–865.

Bazelon, D. L. (1975). A jurist's view of psychiatry. *Journal of Psychiatry and Law, 3,* 175–190.

Bazelon, D. L. (1982). Veils, values, and social responsibility. *American Psychologist, 37,* 115–121.

Beran, N. J., & Toomey, B. G. (1979a). Findings: The community forensic centers. In N. J. Beran & B. G. Toomey (Eds.), *Mentally ill offenders and the criminal justice system: Issues in forensic services* (pp. 119–140). New York: Praeger.

Beran, N. J., & Toomey, B. G. (Eds.). (1979b). *Mentally ill offenders and the criminal justice system: Issues in forensic services.* New York: Praeger.

Bonnie, R. J., & Slobogin, C. (1980). The role of mental health professionals in the criminal process: The case for informed speculation. *Virginia Law Review, 66,* 427–522.

Campbell, D. T., & Stanley, J. C. (1963). *Experimental and quasi-experimental designs for research.* Chicago: Rand McNally.

Carlson, E. W. (1979). Findings: The statewide service delivery system. In N. J. Beran & B. G. Toomey (Eds.), *Mentally ill offenders and the criminal justice system: Issues in forensic services* (pp. 141–174). New York: Praeger.

Churgin, M. J. (1983). The transfer of inmates to mental health facilities: Developments in the law. In J. Monahan & H. J. Steadman (Eds.), *Mentally disordered offenders: Perspectives from law and social science* (pp. 207–232). New York: Plenum Press.

Clingempeel, G., & Reppucci, N. D. (1982). Joint custody after divorce: Major issues and goals for research. *Psychological Bulletin, 91,* 102–127.

Comment. (1979). The psychologist as expert witness: Science in the courtroom? *Maryland Law Review, 38,* 539–621.

Commissioner's Committee on Mental Health and Mental Retardation Forensic Services System. (1982, April). *Final report.* Richmond, VA: Department of Mental Health and Mental Retardation.

160

Davidson, W. S., II, & Saul, J. A. (1982). Youth advocacy in the juvenile court: A clash of paradigms. In G. B. Melton (Ed.), *Legal reforms affecting child and youth services* (pp. 29–42). New York: Haworth.

Department of Justice, Bureau of Justice Statistics. (1983). *Report to the nation on crime and justice: The data.* Washington, DC: U.S. Government Printing Office.

Dix, G. (1971). Psychological abnormality as a factor in grading criminal liability: Diminished capacity, diminished responsibility and the like. *Journal of Criminal Law, Criminology & Political Science, 62,* 313–334.

Dix, G. E., & Poythress, N. G., Jr. (1981). Propriety of medical dominance of forensic mental health practice: The empirical evidence. *Arizona Law Review, 23,* 961–989.

Dowell, D. A., & Ciarlo, J. A. (1983). Overview of the Community Mental Health Centers Program from an evaluation perspective. *Community Mental Health Journal, 19,* 95–125.

Federal Judicial Center. (1981). *Experimentation in the law.* Washington, DC: Author.

Forensic Evaluation Training and Research Center. (1982). *Final report on House Joint Resolution No. 22.* Charlottesville: University of Virginia, Institute of Law, Psychiatry and Public Policy.

Goffman, E. (1961). *Asylums.* New York: Doubleday.

Golding, S. L., Roesch, R., & Schreiber, J. (in press). Assessment and conceptualization of competency to stand trial: Preliminary data on the Interdisciplinary Fitness Interview. *Law and Human Behavior.*

Goldstein, A. (1967). *The insanity defense.* New Haven and London: Yale University Press.

Goldstein, J., Freud, A., & Solnit, A. J. (1973). *Beyond the best interests of the child.* New York: Free Press.

Goldstein, M. S. (1979). The sociology of mental health and illness. *Annual Review of Sociology, 5,* 381–409.

Grisso, T., Sales, B. D., & Bayless, S. (1982). Law-related courses and programs in graduate psychology departments. *American Psychologist, 37,* 267–278.

Group for the Advancement of Psychiatry. (1983). *Community psychiatry: A reappraisal.* New York: Mental Health Materials Center.

Hartstone, E., Steadman, H. J., & Monahan, J. (1982). *Vitek* and beyond: The empirical context of prison-to-hospital transfers. *Law and Contemporary Problems, 45,* 125–136.

Hastings, D. A., & Bonnie, R. J. (1981). A survey of pretrial psychiatric evaluations in Richmond, Virginia. *Developments in Mental Health Law, 1,* 9–12.

Hetherington, E. M., & Martin, B. (1979). Family interaction. In H. C. Quay & J. S. Werry (Eds.), *Psychopathological disorders of childhood* (2nd ed., pp. 247–302). New York: Wiley.

Hiday, V. A. (1977). Reformed commitment procedures: An empirical study in the courtroom. *Law and Society Review, 11,* 651–666.

Hiday, V. A. (1981). Court discretion: Application of the dangerousness standard in civil commitment. *Law and Human Behavior, 5,* 275–289.

Janis, N. R. (1974). Incompetency commitment: The need for procedural safeguards and a proposed statutory scheme. *Catholic University Law Review, 23,* 720–743.

Kiesler, C. A. (1982a). Mental hospitals and alternative care: Noninstitutionalization as potential public policy for mental patients. *American Psychologist, 37,* 349–360.

Kiesler, C. A. (1982b). Public and professional myths about mental hospitalization: An empirical reassessment of policy-related beliefs. *American Psychologist, 37,* 1323–1339.

Laben, J. K., Kashgarian, M., Nessa, D. B., & Spencer, L. D. (1977). Reform from the inside: Mental health center evaluations of competency to stand trial. *Journal of Community Psychology, 5,* 52–62.

Laben, J. K., & Spencer, L. D. (1976). Decentralization of forensic services. *Community Mental Health Journal, 12,* 405–414.

Laboratory of Community Psychiatry. (1974). *Competency to stand trial and mental illness.* New York: Aronson.

Langsley, D. G., & Barter, J. T. (1983). Psychiatric roles in the community mental health center. *Hospital and Community Psychiatry, 34,* 729–733.

Langsley, D. G., & Robinowitz, C. B. (1979). Psychiatric manpower: An overview. *Hospital and Community Psychiatry, 30,* 749–755.

Liss, M. B., & Weinberger, L. E. (1983, October). *Psychologists' knowledge of mental health laws, or I didn't know I was legally responsible for that.* Paper presented at the meeting of the American Psychology-Law Society, Chicago.

Lowery, C. R. (1981). Child custody decisions in divorce proceedings: A survey of judges. *Professional Psychology, 12,* 492–498.

Marx, A. J., Test, M. A., & Stein, C. I. (1973). Extrahospital management of severe mental illness. *Archives of General Psychiatry, 29,* 505–511.

McCall, P. (1979). *Virginia forensic hospital study.* Unpublished Master of Law thesis, University of Virginia, Charlottesville.

McEwen, C. A. (1980). Continuities in the study of total and nontotal institutions. *Annual Review of Sociology, 6,* 143–185.

Melton, G. B. (1981). Effects of a state law permitting minors to consent to psychotherapy. *Professional Psychology, 12,* 647–654.

Melton, G. B. (1983a). Community psychology and rural legal systems. In A. W. Childs & G. B. Melton (Eds.), *Rural psychology* (pp. 359–380). New York: Plenum Press.

Melton, G. B. (1983b). Training in psychology and law: A directory. *Division of Psychology and Law Newsletter, 3*(3), 1–5.

Melton, G. B. (1983c). *Child advocacy: Psychological issues and interventions.* New York: Plenum.

Melton, G. B. (1983d). Community psychology and rural legal systems. In A. W. Childs & G. B. Melton (Eds.), *Rural psychology.* New York: Plenum Press.

Melton, G. B. (1984). Developmental psychology and the law: The state of the art. *Journal of Family Law, 22,* 445–482.

Melton, G. B. (in press). Organized psychology and legal policymaking: Involvement in the post-*Hinckley* debate. *Professional Psychology: Research and Practice.*

162

Melton, G. B., Petrila, J., Poythress, N. G., Jr., & Slobogin, C. (in press). *Psychological evaluations for the courts: A handbook for mental health professionals and the lawyers.* New York: Guilford Press.

Monahan, J. (1973). Abolish the insanity defense? Not yet. *Rutgers Law Review, 26,* 719–740.

Monahan, J. (1981). *The clinical prediction of violent behavior.* Beverly Hills, CA: Sage.

Monahan, J., Davis, S. K., Hartstone, E., & Steadman, H. J. (1983). Prisoners transferred to mental hospitals. In J. Monahan & H. J. Steadman (Eds.), *Mentally disordered offenders: Perspectives from law and social science* (pp. 233–244). New York: Plenum Press.

Morse, S. J. (1978). Crazy behavior, morals, and science. *Southern California Law Review, 51,* 527–653.

Morse, S. J. (1982a). A preference for liberty: The case against involuntary commitment of the mentally disordered. *California Law Review, 70,* 54–106.

Morse, S. J. (1982b). Failed explanations and criminal responsibility: Experts and the unconscious. *Virginia Law Review, 68,* 971–1084.

Morse, S. J. (1982c). Reforming expert testimony: An open response from the tower (and the trenches). *Law and Human Behavior, 6,* 45–49.

Nejelski, P. (1976). Diversion: Unleashing the hound of heaven? In M. K. Rosenheim (Ed.), *Pursuing justice for the child* (pp. 94–118). Chicago: University of Chicago Press.

Ozarin, L. D. (1982). Federal perspectives: The activities of the National Institute of Mental Health in relation to rural mental health services. In P. A. Keller & J. D. Murray (Eds.), *Handbook of rural community mental health* (pp. 158–167). New York: Human Sciences Press.

Pasewark, R. A., & Pantle, M. L. (1979). Insanity plea: Legislator's view. *American Journal of Psychiatry, 136,* 222–223.

Pasewark, R. A., & Seidenzahl, D. (1980). Opinions concerning the insanity plea and criminality among mental patients. *Bulletin of the American Academy of Psychiatry and Law, 8,* 199–202.

Perry, G. S., & Melton, G. B. (1984). Precedential value of judicial notice of social facts: *Parham* as an example. *Journal of Family Law, 22,* 633–676.

Petrella, R. C., & Poythress, N. G., Jr. (1983). The quality of forensic evaluations: An interdisciplinary study. *Journal of Consulting and Clinical Psychology, 51,* 76–85.

Petrila, J. (1981). Forensic psychiatry and community mental health. *Developments in Mental Health Law, 1,* 1–4.

Petrila, J. (1982). The insanity defense and other mental health dispositions in Missouri. *International Journal of Law and Psychiatry, 5,* 81–101.

Petrila, J. P., & Hedlund, J. L. (1983). A computer-supported information system for forensic services. *Hospital and Community Psychiatry, 34,* 451–454.

Poythress, N. G., Jr. (1978). Psychiatric expertise in civil commitment: Training attorneys to cope with expert testimony. *Law and Human Behavior, 2,* 1–23.

Poythress, N. G., Jr. (1982a). Concerning reform in expert testimony: An open letter from a practicing psychologist. *Law and Human Behavior, 6,* 39–45.

Poythress, N. G., Jr. (1982b). *Conflicting postures for mental health expert witnesses: Prevailing attitudes of trial court judges.* Unpublished manuscript, Center for Forensic Psychiatry, Ann Arbor, MI.

Poythress, N. G., Jr. (1983). Psychological issues in criminal proceedings: Judicial preference regarding expert testimony. *Criminal Justice and Behavior, 10,* 175–194.

Poythress, N. G., Jr., & Stock, H. V. (1980). Competency to stand trial: A historical review and some new data. *Journal of Psychiatry and Law, 8,* 131–146.

Reppucci, N. D., & Saunders, J. T. (1983). Focal issues for institutional change. *Professional Psychology: Research and Practice, 14,* 514–528.

Richards, J. M., Jr., & Gottfredson, G. D. (1978). Geographic distribution of U.S. psychologists: A human ecological analysis. *American Psychologist, 33,* 1–9.

Roesch, R. (1978). A brief, immediate screening interview to determine competency to stand trial: A feasibility study. *Criminal Justice and Behavior, 5,* 241–248.

Roesch, R. (1979). Determining competency to stand trial: An examination of evaluation procedures in an institutional setting. *Journal of Consulting and Clinical Psychology, 47,* 542–550.

Roesch, R., & Golding, S. L. (1978). Legal and judicial interpretation of competency to stand trial statutes and procedures. *Criminology, 16,* 420–429.

Roesch, R., & Golding, S. L. (1979). Treatment and disposition of defendants found incompetent to stand trial: A review and a proposal. *International Journal of Law and Psychiatry, 2,* 349–370.

Roesch, R., & Golding, S. L. (1980). *Competency to stand trial.* Urbana: University of Illinois Press.

Rogers, J. L., & Bloom, J. D. (1982). Characteristics of persons committed to Oregon's Psychiatric Security Review Board. *Bulletin of the American Academy of Psychiatry and Law, 10,* 155–164.

Roth, D. (1979). Community-based mental health services for the criminal justice system: The Ohio experience. In N. J. Beran & B. G. Toomey (Eds.), *Mentally ill offenders and the criminal justice system: Issues in forensic services* (pp. 103–106). New York: Praeger.

Runck, B. (1983). NIMH report: Study of 43 jails shows mental health services and inmate safety are compatible. *Hospital and Community Psychiatry, 34,* 1007–1008.

Ryan, J. P., Ashman, A., Sales, B. D., & Shane-DuBow, S. (1980). *American trial judges.* New York: Free Press.

Saks, M. J., & Baron, C. H. (Eds.) (1980). *The use/nonuse/misuse of applied social research in the courts.* Cambridge, MA: Abt Books.

Saks, M. J., & Kidd, R. (1980). Human information processing and adjudication: Trial by heuristics. *Law and Society Review, 15,* 123–160.

Slobogin, C. (1982). *Estelle v. Smith:* The constitutional contours of the forensic evaluation. *Emory Law Journal, 31,* 71–138.

Slobogin, C., Melton, G. B., & Showalter, C. R. (1984). The feasibility of a brief evaluation of mental state at the time of the offense. *Law and Human Behavior, 8,* 305–320.

Steadman, H. J., & Hartstone, E. (1983). Defendants incompetent to stand trial. In J. Monahan & H. J. Steadman (Eds.), *Mentally disordered offenders: Perspectives from law and social science* (pp. 39–62). New York: Plenum Press.

Steadman, H. J., Monahan, J., Hartstone, E., Davis, S. K., & Robbins, C. (1982). Mentally disordered offenders: A national survey of patients and facilities. *Law and Human Behavior, 6,* 31–38.

Steinberg, M. I. (1978). Summary commitment of defendants incompetent to stand trial. *Saint Louis University Law Journal, 22,* 1–24.

Stier, S. D., & Stoebe, K. J. (1979). Involuntary hospitalization of the mentally ill in Iowa: The failure of the 1975 legislation. *Iowa Law Review, 64,* 1284–1458.

Stone, A. (1975). *Mental health and law: A system in transition.* Washington, DC: National Institute of Mental Health.

Stone, A. (1982). Psychiatric abuse and legal reform: Two ways to make a bad situation worse. *International Journal of Law and Psychiatry, 5,* 9–28.

Swigert, V. L., & Farrell, R. A. (1980). Speedy trial and the legal process. *Law and Human Behavior, 4,* 135–145.

Task Force on the Role of Psychology in the Criminal Justice System. (1978). Report. *American Psychologist, 33,* 1099–1113.

Thibaut, J., & Walker, L. (1978). A theory of procedure. *California Law Review, 66,* 541–566.

Torrey, E. F., & Taylor, R. L. (1973). Cheap labor frcm foreign countries. *American Journal of Psychiatry, 130,* 428–433.

Tribe, L. H. (1970). An ounce of detention: Preventive justice in the world of John Mitchell. *Virginia Law Review, 56,* 371–407.

Warren, C. A. B. (1977). Involuntary civil commitment for mental disorder: The application of California's Lanterman-Petris-Short Act. *Law and Society Review, 11,* 629–650.

Wasby, S. L. (1976). *Small town police and the Supreme Court: Hearing the word.* Lexington, MA: Lexington Books.

Whitebread, C. H. (1980). *Criminal procedure: An analysis of constitutional cases and concepts.* Mineola, NY: Foundation Press.

Winick, B. J. (1983). Incompetency to stand trial: Developments in the law. In J. Monahan & H. J. Steadman (Eds.), *Mentally disordered offenders: Perspectives from law and social science* (pp. 3–38). New York: Plenum Press.

Woy, J. R., Wasserman, D. B., & Weiner-Pomerantz, R. (1981). Community mental health centers: Movement away from the model. *Community Mental Health Journal, 17,* 265–276.

Subject Index

Author Index

American Bar Association, 7, 11, 12, 44, 114, 119, 121
American Psychiatric Association, 44, 95
American Psychological Association, 57, 117
Arenella, P., 95
Ashman, J. P., 69–72

Baron, C. H., 78
Barter, J. T., 85
Bayless, S., 118
Bazelon, D. L., 44, 56, 95
Beran, N. J., 6, 16, 17
Bloom, J. D., 114 n. 5
Bonnie, R. J., 1, 11, 44, 95, 116

Campbell, D. T., 20, 23–24
Carlson, E. W., 17
Churgin, M. J., 119
Ciarlo, J. A., 125
Clingempeel, G., 77
Commissioner's Committee, 18, 19, 85, 101, 102

Davidson, W. S., II, 85
Davis, S. K., 4, 119, 123
Department of Justice, 7
Dix, G., 15, 85, 95, 98, 121
Dowell, D. A., 125

Farrell, R. A., 8
Federal Judicial Center, 20, 21
Forensic Evaluation Training and Research Center, 16
Freud, A., 77

Goffman, E., 8
Golding, S. L., 3, 10, 11, 13, 56, 77, 97, 116, 117
Goldstein, J., 77
Goldstein, M. S., 8, 95
Gottfredson, G. D., 15, 116
Grisso, T., 118
Group for the Advancement of Psychiatry, 85

Hartstone, E., 4, 117, 119, 123
Hastings, D. A., 11, 116
Hedlund, J. L., 124
Hetherington, E. M., 76
Hiday, V. A., 77

Janis, N. R., 7

Kashgarian, M., 6, 9, 10, 16, 17, 18, 38
Kidd, R., 108
Kiesler, C. A., 14, 124

Laben, J. K., 6, 9, 10, 16, 17, 18, 38
Laboratory of Community Psychiatry, 13
Langsley, D. G., 15, 85, 116
Liss, M. B., 119
Lowery, C. R., 77

Martin, B., 76
Marx, A. J., 14
McCall, P., 10, 18, 38, 89
McEwen, C. A., 8
Melton, G. B., 1, 2, 3, 10, 12, 13, 38, 44, 45, 77, 78, 85, 93, 97, 115, 117, 118, 119, 121

168

Table of Cases